BUDDHIST PSYCHOLOGY
AND COGNITIVE-BEHAVIORAL THERAPY

Also Available

Emotion Regulation in Psychotherapy:
A Practitioner's Guide
Robert L. Leahy, Dennis Tirch, and Lisa A. Napolitano

Buddhist Psychology and Cognitive-Behavioral Therapy A Clinician's Guide

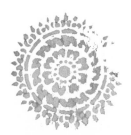

Dennis Tirch
Laura R. Silberstein
Russell L. Kolts

Foreword by Robert L. Leahy

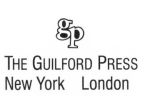

THE GUILFORD PRESS
New York   London

The authors have checked with sources believed to be reliable in their
efforts to provide information that is complete and generally in accord
with the standards of practice that are accepted at the time of publication.
However, in view of the possibility of human error or changes in behavioral,
mental health, or medical sciences, neither the authors, nor the editors and
publisher, nor any other party who has been involved in the preparation or
publication of this work warrants that the information contained herein is
in every respect accurate or complete, and they are not responsible for any
errors or omissions or the results obtained from the use of such information.
Readers are encouraged to confirm the information contained in this book
with other sources.

Library of Congress Cataloging-in-Publication Data

Tirch, Dennis D., 1968–
 Buddhist psychology and cognitive-behavioral therapy : a clinician's guide /
Dennis Tirch, Laura R. Silberstein, Russell L. Kolts.
   pages cm
 Includes bibliographical references and index.
 ISBN 978-1-4625-2324-5 (hardcover)
 1. Buddhism—Psychology. 2. Mindfulness-based cognitive therapy. I. Title.
 BQ4570.P76 T57b2016
 294.3'3615—dc23
                                                            2015013307

To all of my clients, and to the Three Wise Men—
John Tirch, Philip Inwood, and Jeff Peretz
—D. T.

To two Bodhisattvas who happen to be my parents,
Kathy and Stuart Silberstein
—L. R. S.

To Adrienne Isgrigg, whose courageous questions
started me on the path that led me here,
and to Lama Inga Sandvoss, who stewarded me
along the initial part of the journey
—R. L. K.

About the Authors

Dennis Tirch, PhD, is Director of the Center for Compassion Focused Therapy in New York City and Clinical Assistant Professor in the Department of Psychiatry at Weill Cornell Medical College. He is an associate editor of the *Journal of Contextual Behavioral Science* and president of the Compassionate Mind Foundation USA, which is committed to research and training in compassion-focused therapy (CFT). Dr. Tirch serves as president of the New York City Cognitive Behavioral Therapy (CBT) Association and president emeritus of the New York City chapter of the Association for Contextual Behavioral Science (ACBS), and is a Diplomate and Fellow of the Academy of Cognitive Therapy. He provides training internationally for clinicians and researchers and is the author of numerous books, chapters, and peer-reviewed articles on CBT, CFT, acceptance and commitment therapy (ACT), and Buddhist psychology principles.

Laura R. Silberstein, PsyD, is Associate Director of the Center for Compassion Focused Therapy and a consulting psychologist at Memorial Sloan Kettering Cancer Center in New York City. She is also Adjunct Assistant Professor at Albert Einstein College of Medicine of Yeshiva University. Dr. Silberstein is a clinical supervisor and CFT trainer who presents internationally on mindfulness and compassion and is coauthor (with Dennis Tirch and Benjamin Schoendorff) of *The ACT Practitioner's Guide to the Science of Compassion.* She is a founder and executive board member of the New York City chapter of the ACBS and the

Compassionate Mind Foundation USA. Her research interests include psychological flexibility and emotions as well as CFT for anxiety and depression.

Russell L. Kolts, PhD, is Professor of Psychology at Eastern Washington University in Cheney, Washington. Dr. Kolts has authored or coauthored numerous scholarly articles and books, including *An Open-Hearted Life: Transformative Lessons for Compassionate Living from a Clinical Psychologist and a Buddhist Nun* (with Thubten Chodron). He has pioneered the application of CFT to the treatment of problematic anger, regularly conducts trainings and workshops on CFT, and is a board member of the Compassionate Mind Foundation USA.

Foreword

In 2005 I was in Goteborg, Sweden, for the International Conference of Cognitive Psychotherapy, sponsored by the International Association for Cognitive Psychotherapy, of which I was the president. The day before the official program we had Aaron Beck, the founder of cognitive therapy, and the Dalai Lama, the spokesperson for many Buddhists, engage in a dialogue in front of a packed audience. This was an extraordinary event, and the spirit and wisdom of that dialogue pervaded the rest of the conference. As it turned out, Beck had been a practitioner of mindfulness meditation for years, and the Dalai Lama had been an admirer of Beck's cognitive therapy. Beck described how the cognitive therapist asks the client to stand back and observe his or her thoughts and to consider that a thought is not the same thing as reality. And, then, the cognitive therapist asks the client to examine the implications of that thought, the evidence for the thought, and the value of an alternative way of thinking. The Dalai Lama enthusiastically endorsed this as consistent with the Buddhist approach, and the two of them seemed to bond on an intellectual and personal level. In November 2014 a number of us in the cognitive therapy field (e.g., David Clark from the University of Oxford, Stefan Hofmann from Boston University, Judith Beck and Rob DeRubeis from the University of Pennsylvania, Steve Hollon from Vanderbilt University, and Christine Padesky from the Center for Cognitive Therapy) met with Beck in his apartment in Philadelphia. He shared with us the story of the lunch in his home where the Dalai Lama had visited him recently and where they shared their common interest.

This book by Dennis Tirch, Laura R. Silberstein, and Russell L. Kolts is consistent with that bridge between these two great traditions:

Buddhist wisdom and cognitive-behavioral therapy (CBT). What is really unique about this book is the scholarly and detailed description of how Buddhism views the important concepts of reality, impermanence, mindfulness, acceptance, compassion, self, and loving-kindness, and how to engage in the practices that help advance a more meaningful and more complete life. There is much here for the reader from which to learn, not only the historical references and parallels, but also the excellent examples of what to say and what to do with one's clients. There is also far-reaching coverage in this book of why these techniques would be of value.

Of course, within the CBT movement there are many different schools of thought: the Beckian approach, behavioral activation, acceptance and commitment therapy, dialectical behavior therapy, mindfulness-based cognitive therapy, compassion-focused therapy, and others. Some of us disagree with the importance of certain techniques or the assumptions guiding the work that some scholars and clinicians do. That is a natural consequence of an active and open intellectual enterprise. I can tell you that I personally am happy to use anything that works. So I use all of them—but at different times, for different problems, with different clients. I guess I must be practicing flexibility.

But each of these approaches can be related to some aspects of Buddhism. I'm not suggesting that Buddhism necessarily leads to Beckian therapy or to acceptance and commitment therapy, but that Buddhism may add to our understanding of those approaches and place them within a much larger historical context. In reading this book, I came away with a greater appreciation of the wisdom of Buddhism and for the authors who have worked hard to make this important volume clear, informative, practical, and accessible. They are to be commended for their excellent work, and we are fortunate to have that now within our hands.

As a final thought, I recall a few years ago attending my college reunion at Yale. I was sitting there talking to one of my classmates about positive psychology, gratitude, appreciation, and compassion. He looked at me with a twinkle in his eye and said, "Bob, I think some people were talking about this over 2,000 years ago."

I guess we continue to learn what others have already known.

ROBERT L. LEAHY, PHD
Director, American Institute for Cognitive Therapy
Clinical Professor of Psychology,
Department of Psychiatry,
Weill Cornell Medical College

Acknowledgments

My deep appreciation and respect goes out to my wise and compassionate coauthors, Laura and Russell. Over the last 4 years, Laura, you have been my partner on a journey into a new approach to life together, and the writing of this book has been the center of this period of inner and outer work. As we complete this work, I look forward to new beginnings together. Russell, your trust and courage made this book possible. It is an honor, my friend, to have completed this book with you.

Thanks to our dedicated, wise, and clever editors at The Guilford Press, Jim Nageotte and Jane Keislar. Jim, your vision has been essential to creating this book. Jane, your presence, patience, and precision helped us so much. Warm wishes go out to everyone at Guilford who has been a part of this work.

I would like to acknowledge the mentors whom I have been blessed to know, including Robert Leahy, Paul Gilbert, Paul Genki Kahn, Robert Fripp, Kelly Wilson, Steven C. Hayes, Richard Amodio, Lillian Firestone, Michael Hughes, Jim Campilongo, Tony Geballe, and Stephen K. Hayes. Bob Leahy has been especially instrumental in helping this book become a reality. Thanks, Bob, for writing the Foreword too.

My gratitude goes out to all of my trusted colleagues, especially Chris Irons, Martin Brock, Laura Oliff, Poonam Melwani, Louise McHugh, Russ Harris, Benjamin Schoendorff, Robyn Walser, M. Joann Wright, Aisling Curtin, Nanni Presti, Louise Hayes, Christine Braehler, Mia Sage, Richard Sears, Yotam Heineberg, Kristin Neff, Meredith Rayner, Margherita Gurrieri, Sonja Batten, Mark Sisti, Tara Deliberto,

Chris Germer, Brian Pilecki, Ross White, Frank Bond, Emily Sandoz, Christian Chan, Bruce Hubbard, Mike Femenella, Nic Hooper, Tobyn Bell, Trent Codd III, and Zindel Segal.

Laura's family, the Silbersteins, were also a great source of strength during our work. I would like to thank my wonderful mother and family, especially my brother, John, and his miraculously supportive wife and children. I would like to acknowledge the help and support of our friends as we prepared this book, particularly Mark and Elizabeth Christensen and Philip Inwood. Also, I want to send good wishes to all of the clients who have walked this compassionate path with us over the years.

Finally, I would like to express my gratitude to our spiritual ancestors, who are innumerable and represent the evolution that we hold so dear. For our purposes today, I would like to acknowledge, with deep love and respect, Shakyamuni Buddha, Chogyam Trungpa Rinpoche, John G. Bennett, Shunryu Suzuki, George Ivanovich Gurdjieff, and Keith Richards for the win. . . .

—D. T.

The path that led to the completion of this book would never have been possible without the support and guidance of many like-minded and like-hearted people. I am honored and grateful to have the chance to acknowledge these contributors and guides, in particular coauthors Dennis Tirch and Russell Kolts. Not enough could be said to express my appreciation and admiration for these two individuals and the work they do. Russ, your profound warmth, empathy, kindness, and enthusiasm are a source of wonder, motivation, and encouragement for me. Dennis, thank you for your partnership, friendship, and acceptance, and for a shared quest for "knowing."

I would also like to express my appreciation and gratitude to those individuals who have become my touchstones in this work and beyond. To my sister, Erica, thank you for showing me the grace and precision in being sensitive to others and teaching me that unrelenting strength can come with a desire to change the world. To my parents, your tacit and explicit life lessons gave me courage, curiosity, and perspective, and I am forever grateful.

Thank you to all of those who took the time and patience to teach and learn with me, including Paul Gilbert, Thomas Bein, Robert Leahy, Lata McGinn, James Cardinale, Robert Woolfolk, Leslie Allen, Shara Sand, Kelly Wilson, Steven Hayes, Jack Kornfield, Sharon Salzberg, Chris Irons, Chris Germer, Kristin Neff, Tom Borkovec, Brad Richards,

Linda Dimeff, Lauren Whitelaw, and Jeff Young. There are many groups and communities to whom I am forever grateful to call home and family, including the Fritz, Young, Kondo, Tirch, Mann, Reichenbach, ACBS, ACT-NYCE, CFT, CBT, DBT, and OMEGA families. Thank you all for creating contexts where loving-kindness, compassion, sympathetic joy, and equanimity are possible.

—L. R. S.

First and foremost, I would like to acknowledge my wonderful coauthors, Dennis Tirch and Laura Silberstein. Without your vision and dedication, this book would not have been possible. More importantly, your kindness, wisdom, commitment, and friendship inspire me on a daily basis. I would also like to thank my wife, Lisa Koch, my son, Dylan Kolts, and my parents, John and Mary Kolts, whose constant support lifts my spirits and allows me to contribute to projects such as this one.

The support from my colleagues and community at Eastern Washington University has been invaluable, as have my connections with my dear friends and colleagues in the compassion-focused therapy community, including Paul Gilbert and the Gilbert family, Dennis and Laura, Chris Irons and Korina Ioannou, Deborah Lee, Mary Welford, Michelle Cree, Lynn Henderson, Tobyn Bell, Kate Lucre, Christine Braehler, Fiona Ashworth, Neil Clapton, Ken Goss, and many others. All of you have provided me with the support, encouragement, and friendship that create the perfect conditions for doing this work. Thanks, friends.

—R. L. K.

Contents

Purchasers of this book can download
audio files of the guided meditations
from *www.guilford.com/tirch-materials*
for personal use or use with individual clients.

BUDDHIST PSYCHOLOGY
AND COGNITIVE-BEHAVIORAL THERAPY

Introduction to the Functional Relationship between Buddhist Psychology and Cognitive-Behavioral Therapy

The past should not be followed after,
And the future not desired.
What is past is dead and gone,
And the future is yet to come.

But whoever gains insight into things
Presently arisen in the here and now,
Knowing them, unmoved, unshaken—
Let him cultivate that insight.
—THE BUDDHA, *Majjhima Nikaya* 3.187

All the things that you love are going to change; you're going to lose them one way or another. It makes them all the more precious.
—JEFF BRIDGES and ROSHI BERNIE GLASSMAN,
The Dude and the Zen Master

Throughout history, human beings have consistently worked to develop effective ways to alleviate their suffering. In different eras, the paradigms of the day have led to a diversity of spiritual and secular techniques designed to quiet the turbulence of the mind, and to heal our emotional

1

and physical pain. From shamanistic rituals designed to evoke helpful spirits, to Catholic rites of confession; from Freudian psychoanalysis to functional magnetic resonance imaging of the brain, the question of human suffering consistently has inspired technological innovation and philosophical questions (Gilbert, 1989; Moyers, 1993; Woolfolk, 1998). Despite how difficult life is, we human beings keep striving to make things more workable, to be happier, and make life ever more livable, with a heartfelt tenacity in the face of its difficulties or tragedies. Some prescientific methods, such as Zen meditation, have endured for centuries, with millions of people reporting that these practices have enhanced their lives, and lessened their burden. Other techniques based in scientific research, such as cognitive-behavioral therapy (CBT), may only be decades old, but nevertheless present us with a particular advantage. The scientific method allows us to refine and specify our psychological technologies. As a result, we can test and replicate the degree to which particular processes and procedures are able to predict and influence human behavior (Barnes-Holmes, Hayes, Barnes-Holmes, & Roche, 2002; Hawton, Salkovskis, Kirk, & Clark, 1989; Skinner, 1953). In this way, we can hone interventions that provide us with a reliable and practical approach to the question of human suffering. Our cognitive and behaviorial therapy techniques have been thoroughly empirically supported and widely disseminated, helping people throughout the world to liberate themselves from psychological distress. As this research proceeds, methods become refined, with new techniques emerging and less useful methods being discarded. In this way, science has accelerated our understanding of suffering and how to respond to it.

Furthermore, as our understanding of evidence-based psychotherapies and ancient contemplative practices has deepened, certain commonalities have emerged that suggest possibilities for integration of cognitive and behavioral methods and meditative practices. Such integration of ancient wisdom traditions and research-based psychotherapies is generating new directions for applied psychological science.

This book aims to provide a comprehensive introduction to applied Buddhist psychology for CBT practitioners. We wish to help clarify available points of consideration in the integration of Buddhist psychology and CBT, perhaps creating a few new possibilities for the clinician. Further applications and adaptation of the evidence-based principles in Buddhist psychology and CBT are waiting to be undertaken. By clarifying these foundations and practices, we hope to share in this evolutionary process with our readers and our communities.

CBT AND BUDDHIST PSYCHOLOGY IN CONCEPT AND PRACTICE

This book focuses on two effective, widely disseminated and increasingly well-researched methods: CBT and Buddhist psychology. Rather than consisting of a single, unified model of mental functioning, the term "CBT" represents a community of empirically supported treatments, which currently are recognized as the "gold-standard" approach to psychotherapy, in terms of efficacy research. This recognition appears to be due to the emphasis within CBT on scientific methods and evidence-based practices (Baker, McFall, & Shoham, 2009). Taken as a whole, CBT approaches have several hundred randomized controlled trials supporting their effectiveness for a wide range of psychological problems. The evidence is particularly strong for cognitive therapy (Butler, Chapman, Forman, & Beck, 2006) and CBT for anxiety disorders (Barlow, 2004), which have an outstanding track record for outcome research. Additionally, the processes involved in cognitive and behavioral therapies are often linked to basic experimental research (Ruiz, 2010; Alford & Beck, 1998), and research that indicates that treatment processes actively mediate significant change in therapy outcomes. This emphasis on empirically supported processes and mediation research has been particularly prevalent within the acceptance and commitment therapy (ACT) literature (Hayes, Strosahl, & Wilson, 2011). CBT is host to a significant number of treatment models and scientific theories that have both significant similarities and evolving differences in language, technique, or philosophy. These changes emerge through the ongoing work of a global scientific community, consisting of active research programs and thousands of clinicians employing evidence-based techniques. At this point, the vast range of CBT theories and models "have been applied to the full range of human experiences" (Herbert & Forman, 2011, p. 1), with the aim of reducing mental illness and increasing well-being.

"Buddhist psychology," as we use the term here, refers to both a tradition of psychological techniques and an applied philosophy of mind, that have been used within Buddhism for at least 2,600 years to help people liberate themselves from suffering. Buddhism, in its essence, is not a religion in the same way that any of the other global, theistic, and spiritual traditions are. Although culturally situated lineages of Buddhist teaching have espoused beliefs in reincarnation or other spiritual phenomena, there are no claims made in Buddhist psychology or in the teachings of the historical Buddha concerning the existence of a God, life after death, or the presence of a soul. Thus, Buddhism is an ongoing incomplete endeavor with many branches and schools of thought just as is Western science and experimentation.

At times, voices in the cultural discussion may question whether researchers and clinicians ought to be applying elements of religion to a scientific process. This argument would be important and valid if we were discussing the adoption of mystical assumptions in the absence of scientific analysis, experimentation, and replication. Furthermore, if we were adopting the assumptions of theistic religions, or asserting the existence of a God, gods, or supernatural entities whose existence is not falsifiable, we would be on very shaky intellectual and ontological ground. However, the integration of Buddhist psychology into the process of the development of a global psychology best suited to the needs of the human condition does none of the above. In the integration of CBT and Buddhist psychology, we are describing an evidence-based appreciation of applied psychological systems for the alleviation of suffering that have emerged cross-culturally and transdiagnostically.

Essentially, applied Buddhist psychology can be viewed as processes of discovery, and individual empiricism. Buddhism emphasizes such empiricism, and Buddhist teachings are only as good as their current validity and reliability (Dalai Lama, 1991). Even the most central teachings are to be examined and not just taken as truth; and if proven wrong through vigorous empirical testing, then they ought to be subject to change and progress (Dalai Lama, 1991). Buddhist psychology teaches not through revelation or blind faith, but through investigation and analysis. Through the observation of experiences, as well as an understanding of cause and effect and the relationship between reality and consciousness, Buddhism offers an alternative way of navigating the human experience.

According to tradition, at some point in the sixth century B.C.E., The Shakyamuni Buddha, once a member of the tribal aristocracy in the western Himalayas, became a serious student of the meditation and philosophical traditions that were practiced on the Indian subcontinent.

At that point in history, numerous techniques of yoga, attention training, and behavioral change methods had been developed throughout the region, within a centuries-old, prescientific tradition that related to spiritual scriptures. The Buddha mastered these methods, and then proceeded to develop an innovative technology for training the mind for liberation from suffering. The Buddha's approach eschewed spiritual and supernatural assumptions, and depended upon individual practices, and pragmatic results. This method became widespread in the region during the time of the Buddha's life, and spread widely after his death. For the next 26 centuries, the method went through a consistent process of rigorous research and development through the practice of millions of Buddhist monks, scholars, and lay practitioners throughout the world. While this process did not follow the sequence prescribed by Western science, Buddhism has contained a form of subjective, pragmatic empiricism, logical analysis, and neurophenomenology (Varela, 1996) throughout its evolution. In the 20th and 21st centuries, the subjective empiricism of earlier Buddhism has begun to merge with the Western scientific tradition, to suggest the possibility of a more refined, scientifically grounded Buddhist psychology.

BEGINNING WHERE YOU ARE

Please take a moment to bring your attention directly to your physical experience, here and now. If it is safe to do so, please close your eyes for a few seconds and take three deep, slow, and full breaths while paying attention to the physical sensations involved in breathing, as much as you can. Then open your eyes and return to the next paragraph.

As you hold the tablet, smartphone, or book that contains these words, you can feel its weight in your hands. You examine patterns of black and white symbols, which confer meaning. This all happens simultaneously, and seemingly effortlessly. You're not likely to be noticing any of that, and you may simply just be aware of the act of reading.

You might just be "hearing" the words you read "in your head." Your attention may have already wandered away from the book to some daydream of tomorrow, or some reminiscence of the past. All of this is a part of your unique human experience of being alive right now. As far as we are aware, no other animal can process all of this at once or have this sort of experience.

This realization leads us to adapt and paraphrase a portion of an ancient series of observations from the original teachings of the historical Buddha, known as the *Dhammapada* (Cleary, 1994; Friedlander, 2009):

- Given how rare it is that the conditions to potentially sustain life might emerge on a planet, isn't it amazing that you are even here in the first place, right now?

- And given how unlikely it is that life would evolve to the level of human consciousness, isn't it quite strange that you would have the ability to think at all, let alone read?

- And when we consider how difficult life on earth has been for so many human beings, and how rare it is to live in a time of relative peace and prosperity, how fortunate are we to be able to communicate through this book, together, here and now?

- If someone were watching over your shoulder just now, he or she would likely witness a human being who is relatively safe and healthy, who is well fed and educated, and who is seeking to learn more about how to help his or her fellow human beings to alleviate their suffering.

- Isn't it worth pausing and appreciating this event, even if just for its remarkable rarity in the known universe?

We know the human brain has more discrete possible connections across its nerve cells than there are stars in the sky, or grains of sand on a beach (Davidson, Jackson, & Kalin, 2000; LeDoux, 2002). The capacity we human beings have for language, thought, pattern recognition, and making comparisons between stimuli is unlike anything demonstrated by other animals. The human capacity to interact with the environment, to adapt, and to create tools for problem solving is awe-inspiring in its efficiency and evolutionary elegance. Beyond this, our potential for wisdom, compassion, and kindness is exceptional. Unlike other species, we have evolved to possess a potential for unconditional love and generosity.

Nonetheless, as you are human, then we also know something rather less heartening about you. We know you are struggling, and we know you are suffering.

We know this because it is the nature of the human mind to suffer and to struggle. Given our typical "day-to-day" human perspective, life can seem consistently out of balance, like the feeling of a wheel that is slightly out of alignment.

Though we live in an era of relative global prosperity, 50% of the general population will suffer from a major psychological disorder over the course of their lives (Kessler et al., 1994; Kessler, Chiu, Demler, & Walters, 2005). Beyond that, millions who don't "earn" such a diagnosis experience problems with addiction or other self-destructive behaviors. Approximately half of us seriously contemplate suicide at some point in our lives (Chiles & Strosahl, 2005). Many experience tragic losses, abuse, neglect, or deprivation. All of us will die. Extreme poverty can be found in the shadow of staggering wealth. Nations fight wars with one another on horrific scales, spreading death, injury, disaster, poverty, and hatred.

Despite the miracle of human consciousness, most of us will experience a chronic "dis-ease" through which our experience will be tainted with some measure of chronic unhappiness and anxious apprehension. This "dis-ease" may be described as "the stress and intrinsic unsatisfactoriness of a life that is always seeking some other state or condition in which to feel fulfilled, complete and happy" (Kabat-Zinn, 2009, p. xxvii). In a sense, the central truth of the human experience is a truth of suffering.

In the midst of all of this struggle and pain, musician and composer Robert Fripp said, "A reasonable person might despair, but hope is unreasonable, and love is stronger than even that." As we observed, over the past several thousand years, wisdom traditions, mind sciences, and meditative disciplines have evolved to point a way out of the cycle of human suffering. As we will discuss together, this path forward involves compassion, wisdom, flexible response patterns, and the capacity to experience distress with courage and clear awareness. While the human condition cannot be avoided, we have no choice but to be human; we do, however, have a choice as to what to do with it. We can search for new answers, new ways of using what is both our gift and our affliction: our human mind. That which is the source of our suffering can also be our salvation.

As we take a closer look at CBT and Buddhist psychology, we find traditions that have evolved in different cultural contexts. However, these traditions share common aims, common techniques, and even elements of a common history. More importantly, CBT and Buddhist psychology are beginning to affect one another's development and perspectives.

Both Buddhist psychology and CBT aim to observe, question, and alleviate the experience of suffering by providing a clearer understanding of reality and creating an effective context to cultivate new approaches to one's struggles and personal development. Both Buddhist psychology and CBT have accessible and powerful contributions to offer one another in the pursuit of shared aims and functions.

From this point forward, at least in the Western world, it may be that CBT and Buddhism are evolving into one another. This turn of events was predicted over a century ago by one of CBT's forerunners, the great American psychologist William James. According to James (1902/2009), Buddhism was the "psychology everybody will be studying 25 years from now." James's prediction was accurate, though he placed the current Buddhist-informed revolution in Western psychology 100 or so years too early.

THE CURRENT AND FUTURE INTEGRATION

Over the course of the last two decades, methods and concepts that have been associated with Buddhism for centuries have become the central focus of much CBT research and development. CBT has been described as undergoing a third wave of innovation (Herbert & Forman, 2011) that has everything to do with a proliferation of methods based in such Buddhist-informed concepts as mindfulness, acceptance, and compassion. To varying degrees, both CBT and Buddhist psychology train people to cultivate a present-moment-focused awareness of our experience, in order to cut through the influence of delusional beliefs and destructive emotions (Dalai Lama, 1991; Kwee, Gergen, & Koshikawa, 2006). Furthermore, both schools of thought employ forms of analytic reasoning to question the merit and believability of distressing thinking, as well as contemplative, experiential techniques to reduce psychological suffering (Baker et al., 2009; Guenther & Kawamura, 1975). This blend of positive psychological change, based both on knowledge and in direct experience, is a primary characteristic of the integration of Buddhist psychology and CBT. Accordingly, throughout this book, we will be providing you with a blend of information and practical exercises. Each of the meditative practices we present to you can be used with patients in therapy. However, you can also use these exercises to deepen your understanding of the concepts we are discussing.

An amazing combination and flow of elements have occurred in the last three decades allowing us to understand more fully what drives our suffering, and how we can develop ever more efficient ways to foster its alleviation. Technological advances in fast and efficient travel, and an exponential acceleration of information technology, have led to a global exchange of ideas, across cultures and philosophical systems. Even just 50 years ago, most of the information on Buddhism and psychology that we have at our fingertips would be literally inaccessible to most people, including most psychologists. Beginning with the 1960s counterculture and expanding with Internet technologies, practices such as yoga, Buddhist meditation, and other philosophies from Eastern religions have pervaded Western medicine and popular culture.

During this same era, several areas of psychological science have experienced major advances that have involved a greater study of Buddhist psychology as a method of addressing psychological problems. For example, computer technology has resulted in much more precise imaging of our brains and neurophysiology. As a result, neuroscientists have more precisely described the ways that emotions, attention, and meditative training are expressed in the brain (Austin, 1999; LeDoux 1996, 1998, 2002; Treadway & Lazar, 2009). In terms of behavioral research, experimental and theoretical advancements in the behavioral analysis of human language have resulted in a new understanding of just how human beings are able to think and communicate. These developments have led to effective new methods for conducting psychotherapy (Hayes, 2004b; Hayes, Villatte, Levin, & Hildebrant, 2011). Advances in evolutionary psychology have illuminated the function and origins of much of what drives our psychological struggle and pain (Gilbert, 1998a, 2001; Kurzban & Leary, 2001; Wilson, 2004). Despite the roots of these movements being deep in the Western scientific tradition, all of these developments have lead researchers and practitioners to place mindfulness, acceptance, and compassion, fundamental elements of a Buddhist approach, at the center of new directions for applied clinical psychology (Goleman, 1991; Kang & Whittingham, 2010).

Following on these trends in science and culture, a wide range of new psychotherapies has emerged in CBT. These new therapies draw upon the most effective and research-proven methods of previous psychotherapies, and expand the CBT tradition through the elaboration of a new understanding of the nature of thinking, feeling, and doing. Beyond even this, these cutting-edge approaches emphasize ways that human beings may establish a new relationship to their experience, through the cultivation of acceptance, mindful awareness of the present moment, and compassion. These therapies, including ACT (Hayes et al., 2011), functional analytic psychotherapy (FAP; Kohlenberg & Tsai, 1991), compassion-focused therapy (CFT; Gilbert, 2009a, 2010a), mindfulness-based stress reduction (MBSR; Kabat-Zinn, 1990), mindfulness-based cognitive therapy (MBCT; Segal, Williams, & Teasdale, 2002), mindfulness-based relapse prevention (MBRP; Marlatt & Donovan, 2005), and dialectical behavior therapy (DBT; Linehan,1993a), have come to define the direction of CBT. Directly and indirectly, Buddhism informs these modalities on the levels of theory and practice (Hayes, 2004b; Kang & Whittenham, 2010). Beyond these cutting-edge innovations, elements of Buddhism may have informed the development of CBT from its inception. For example, according to Albert Ellis, "While Rational Emotive Behavioral Therapy (REBT) highlights the norm of people's dogmatic, fanatical and rigid beliefs, it has *always* favored several aspects of Zen Buddhism as a Modus Vivendi" (Kwee & Ellis, 1998, p. 5; original emphasis). Buddhist models of human psychology have evolved over centuries of devoted contemplation, scholarship, and meditation. They have been recorded in thousands of volumes, which are centuries-old. Some of these texts have yet to be translated into modern or Western languages. This pool of knowledge and analysis of experience is currently being decoded by some of the best and brightest minds in Western intellectual traditions, and interpreted in the light of a global neuroscience initiative. We are beginning to understand the nature of mind from an integral, multicultural perspective, and we are beginning to test and implement methods for freeing the mind from its struggles.

All of this is available to us, for the good of our patients and ourselves. Right now, the sum of Buddhist and Western scientific thought can begin to point us in the direction of personal liberation, the alleviation of suffering, the cultivation of wisdom, and a growing compassionate mode of being. In our everyday life as clinicians, it will be a rare day that a person comes to us with a presenting problem that reads: "Seeking personal liberation." Nevertheless, when we seek to help our clients get out from under the dominance of excessive worries and rumination we are helping them to become free to live bigger, more meaningful lives. When we meet someone with agoraphobia or major depression, who has surrendered the outside world to become a functional prisoner of the four walls of their room, we are helping to alleviate and prevent their ongoing suffering, and to develop the liberating self-compassion that they might need to face their fears and regrets.

Despite the wide proliferation of Buddhist publications, and the exponential growth in meditation and psychotherapy research, what has emerged so far can seem like myriad streams that flow in different directions. It is a quirk of our educational systems that scholars in various areas don't always reach one another with their discoveries. Rather than an ivory tower, the world of academic science may be better compared to an ivory archipelago, as David Sloan Wilson (2007) suggests. Each school of thought, on its own island, may be making great progress in researching an area of inquiry, with a given methodology. Nevertheless, these islands might not communicate in a way that allows for adaptive, prosocial cooperation. Neuroscientists may not be speaking with the behavioral researchers. Psychiatrists may be cut off from individuals who study the social impact of economic forces. Something is lost in this absence of communication. Even within the discipline of psychology, for example, there are isolated pockets of scholarship, so that the right hand of a science might not know what its left hand is doing. How many of us have learned a great deal about a given theoretical approach, for example, psychoanalytic theory, and have remained ignorant of what is happening in an allied modality, such as applied behavioral analysis. We know that for science to advance, it is necessary that scholars and researchers pursue ever more specialized lines of inquiry. Yet this specialization often isolates them from the broader discussion. In a sense, the intellectual, disciplinary archipelago is a side effect of our current educational systems. However, it doesn't have to be like this.

In the midst of the current revolution in psychology and related fields, there are significant efforts to address this side effect, and to bring together many disciplines that examine consciousness and suffering from a cross-cultural point of view. One great example is the work of the Mind and Life Institute (*www.mindandlife.org*), which has brought authorities on Buddhist philosophy, such as His Holiness the Dalai Lama, into discussions with Western physicists, psychologists, and other scientists (1991). Organizations like the Association for Contextual Behavioral Science, the Association for Behavioral and Cognitive Therapies, and the Compassionate Mind Foundation all provide a context where concepts from CBT and Buddhist psychology can be integrated. Nonetheless, we have yet to develop a user-friendly guide to the basics of Buddhist psychology that provides a road map designed for the CBT clinician. Of course, there are huge numbers of publications about the alphabet soup of different cognitive and behavioral therapies (CBT, MBCT, DBT, etc.), but there is more available in Buddhist psychology than has been presented to cognitive behavioral therapists so far.

The adaptation of Buddhist psychology methods to CBT has centered on the concept of mindfulness (DiDonna, 2009). Depending on where and how mindfulness is referenced in the psychotherapy literature, this concept may stand for a process, a procedure, an outcome, a form of training, or even the entirety of Buddhist philosophy. Needless to say, this ambiguity can lead to some measure of confusion. In exploring and clarifying Buddhist psychology for the CBT clinician, we will explore these aspects of mindfulness in some detail. However, we can begin with the elegantly simple definition of mindfulness put forward by Germer, Siegel, and Fulton (2005): *awareness of present experience with acceptance.* "With acceptance" means this kind of awareness includes allowing public or private processes without trying to change or challenge their existence. As we touch on mindfulness in our initial discussion, we can return to this direct, clear, conceptual understanding.

Clinical psychologists target secular aims, and, in many respects, are limited to techniques that are based on empirical evidence. In this way, psychologists are assured that their work is based on scientific grounds, even when inspired by sources from spiritual philosophies. However, something would be lost if we were to turn our back upon the whole of Buddhist philosophy and psychology until such time that each element has been researched, packaged, commodifed, and branded in a Western idiom. As Dimidjian and Linehan (2003, p. 167) have suggested, "It is possible that relinking mindfulness with its spiritual roots may enhance clinical practice." Similarly, Hayes (2002a, p. 105) asserted, "Combining these two great traditions, spirituality and science, promises a leap forward in our understanding of human suffering, but only if psychological scientists keep their eye on the development of a coherent and progressive discipline, not merely the acquisition of a few new clinical maneuvers."

As we encounter Buddhist psychology as behaviorists, cognitive therapists, or researchers in applied psychology, we bring the perspective of the scientific method to Buddhism. In this book, as we explore Buddhist source materials for tools to use in combination with CBT, the alleviation of suffering and the promotion of lives of purpose, meaning, and vitality are our aims, rather than the promotion of a state of "spiritual enlightenment." We will provide examples of CBT and Buddhist techniques that are compatible with evidence-based clinical practice. For example, in Chapter 10 we provide a case conceptualization method and worksheet that is derived from Buddhist concepts and intentions, yet which facilitates the targeted delivery of specific CBT interventions. Ultimately, though, our clinical aims are in complete accord with the teachings of Buddhism, wherein reified supernatural assumptions are to be avoided, and the pursuit of the alleviation of suffering is ever-present. Whatever "enlightenment" may be, it is helpful for this discussion to see it as a description of a frame of mind. This description has been left for us by individuals who have reportedly completed a process of realizing their human potential, through rigorous and stimulating mental training, in the face of great adversity. Whatever enlightenment comes to mean to you is your decision. The mission of the alleviation of human suffering and the promotion of growth is something clinical psychologists and other clinicians share. From this common ground, we can step forward.

CLARIFYING THE PROCESS

In Tibetan Vajrayana Buddhist temples, "butter lamps" (candles) are used that are made of clarified yak butter. This practice probably emerged because yak butter is more readily available than wax in the Himalayas. Yet there is also a symbolic significance to the clarified golden butter that glows in these brass candles. It is taught that, through the process of gradual Buddhist mental training, repeatedly coming into direct contact with the true nature of mind, our struggle with mental illusions dissipates and is clarified. Buddhist teachings describe an illuminated "clear seeing" that emerges through contemplative training that is akin to the clarification of butter. Gradually seeing through cognitive distortions, delusions, and emotionally cloudy perceptions is said to result in an experience of the "clear light" of pure conscious awareness, symbolized by the light glowing through the clear surface of the butter lamp (Baer, 2003).

At this point in the integration of Buddhist psychology and CBT, there is just so much information available, and so many seemingly disparate perspectives on Westernized mindfulness techniques, that it can be hard to clarify the central concepts of Buddhism, and how they might relate to cognitive-behavioral practice. Even for those of us who "do mindfulness" as psychotherapists, the concepts, the body of research, and the intention behind the practices derived from Buddhist psychology can seem confusing and clouded in obscure terminology and cultural baggage.

Importantly, everything in this book is drawn from earlier Buddhist psychology and CBT resources, and our aim is to provide this to you in a new form for your better access and understanding. As there are many concepts that we will be surveying, we have included a very brief Appendix (at the end of the book) that outlines some key concepts. You can think of it as your dharma "cheat sheet" as you come to engage more fully with the concepts in Buddhism that can be readily applied to our clinical work. However, you already possess everything you need to work with the material in this book in meaningful ways. Buddhist psychology holds that all of us are already fully liberated and endlessly wise, but that this wisdom may not be available to us in our current state of affairs. From this point of view, you are already in possession of everything you need to break the cycle of suffering that holds you (and your clients) in place. This may sound a little weird at first, but, from a Buddhist perspective, right now, literally speaking, you are already "perfectly enlightened." You just aren't aware of it yet. The methods presented in the following pages will aim to make you more aware of this natural inner wisdom, in the service of the alleviation of suffering for you and your patients.

Throughout this book, you will encounter a number of experiential exercises and meditations. Derived from Buddhist practice and third-wave cognitive and behaviorial therapies, these practices are meant to both illustrate the concepts we are encountering, and to provide a form of practice that is relevant to clinical practice. These practices may be used with patients, and may be integrated into existing CBT modalities, to enhance training in mindfulness and self-compassion, and to further the aims of the treatment. You will find the practices provided set apart from our text in boxes that highlight each as an experiential exercise. Throughout its history, Buddhism has adapted and grown to better fit with the cultures and human conditions it encountered. Rather than providing a system of orthodox Buddhist practice, which can be found in a variety of sources, this book presents concepts, meditations, and exercises that are particularly relevant to the integrated practice of

Buddhist psychology and CBT. As mentioned, we also encourage you to experiment with these practices as you read through the text. To further this aim, we have provided audio recordings of all of these practices for you at *www.guilford.com/tirch-materials*. You can use these recordings to guide your practice, or work from the descriptions that are here in this book. Most importantly, we invite you to engage with this material experientially, and to use your own clinical wisdom and understanding to bridge into the experiences we discuss.

A First Experiential Step

For just a few minutes, let's step out of the structure of a conventional text, so that we might engage in a small experiential exercise. During this exercise, you will ask yourself a series of mildly provocative questions. There will be many exercises involved in this work you are beginning, so let's think of this as just "one taste" of a new level of engagement with this material. Many readers will recognize this practice as involving a concept from Buddhist psychology known as "mindfulness." If you have some experience with mindfulness, perhaps you might hold your knowledge of mindfulness as lightly as possible, as you approach this practice and all of that which follows. If you have no experience of mindfulness, or are unfamiliar with the term, you can rest assured that the rest of your reading here (as well as a casual stroll through the poster presentations at a CBT conference) will bring you into consistent contact with definitions and descriptions of mindfulness. For now, let's just view this exercise as a quiet, restful, and curious experiment. You might even think of it as a game, if that is helpful. A series of instructions and questions will follow. Later, after you read the questions, as best you can, try not to worry about whether the answers that present themselves to you are "right" or "wrong" or "true" or "false." They are just questions to be encountered, and your reactions are simply to be noticed, with acceptance, moment by moment.

As best you can, try simply to observe and be present with these reactions without judging them. Perhaps you might bring a little curiosity and kindness to the experience.

Guided Instructions

If you are willing, take a moment now, and breathe deeply and naturally in and out of the abdomen. For about 60 seconds after I ask you to begin [a few lines down] allow your eyes to close and just let that breath breathe itself in and out of your body.

Feel your feet on the ground.

Feel your back straight and supported, and feel yourself rooted to the earth like a strong and stable tree, or even a mountain. Take some time to rest in the breath, in a spirit of acceptance and kindness. With each in-breath, you breathe attention and life into your body. With each out-breath, you let go, literally releasing the tension and the air that no longer sustains you, letting go more and more with each exhalation.

After about a minute or two of just being with that breath, simply watching what happens, open your eyes and read the series of questions that follows. Please read each question slowly, and give yourself time to make space for whatever arises in response to the question. Pause and let yourself notice and appreciate the thoughts, feelings, and sensations that unfold before your observation, moment by moment, after each question. Let some time pass, perhaps 10 to 30 seconds between each question. Exhaling, and letting go, move on to the next question. There are no answers. Just watching what happens.

When you are ready, please begin.

If you have taken the time to breathe in silence and approach the words below, please continue.

"What if everything you've learned wasn't exactly wrong, but was founded on an illusion?"

"What if the nature of who you really are is completely different from what you've been taught?"

"What if you found out that you were infinitely and inextricably connected to everything else that exists, and that all perceived separateness was something of a dream?"

"What if a part of you already knows this, and that part connects with the 'rightness' of these words, in the present moment, as you read this book, right now?"

"What if all things as we know them revealed themselves to be impermanent?"

"What would that mean for you? What would that say about your freedom?"

"What if you could naturally, precisely, and relaxedly draw your attention to the flow of your conscious experience, on purpose, with clear seeing . . .

and . . . in this way, you could come to see thoughts as thoughts, emotions as emotions, sensations as sensations,

and. . . . find an experience of self that is beyond identification with anything in particular?"

"What if, from that perspective, you could wake up to the reality of what is happening right now, fully and deeply, without defense, experiencing the present moment, as best you can, and choose to take actions that are meaningful and purposeful to you, moment by moment?"

"What would that mean for your grocery shopping? For your parenting? For your home repair budget?"

"How can you be fully awake and alive, abiding in absolute reality, while you attend to the relative reality that you are co-creating right here and right now?"

"How is it that this makes sense to you?"

"How is it that it doesn't make sense?"

Now that our first exercise is complete, we can let it go, with a deep, cleansing exhalation. When you have completed this book, all of the above questions might seem pretty simple and straightforward. Then again, they may remain a complete mystery. Maybe both situations will be equally true. If you have experience with ACT, DBT, Zen, mindfulness, or yoga philosophy, some of this may be quite familiar already. Whatever your background, the aim of this book is to link the abstract with the precise, and spiritual concepts with the scientific method. You will learn how an integration of Buddhist psychology and CBT allows us to shift our perspective in adaptive ways, and to become unstuck from our habitual patterns of perception and action.

For now, take a moment to give yourself some credit for engaging with this first exercise, and, as you consciously exhale, try to let any of the questions or their potential answers go. This little introductory exercise is the first of many that we will outline and explain in far greater detail. You will find these exercises interspersed throughout the text. We would encourage you to actually engage in these practices, availing yourself of the downloadable guided practices when you can. Your understanding of the concepts here, and your use of the practical techniques that follow, will allow you to bring many potentially powerful elements of Buddhist psychology to your practice of cognitive and behavioral psychotherapy, in ways that are consistent with the state of the art of the CBT process and outcome research.

If you are a student, a researcher, or a clinician who is involved in practice-based research, we would encourage you to pay close attention to the questions that arise for you as you read this book. This is a time of exploration and expansion for the integration of CBT and Buddhist psychology. As such, the more we can identify further questions and lines of study, the better off we are. As scientist practitioners, our shared mission is to frame these questions in testable, scientific ways. In doing so, and by sharing these questions with our community, we can spur further research and reflection, driving the science and practice of the alleviation of human suffering ever forward.

In a rough approximation of one of His Holiness the Dalai Lama's suggestions, if the techniques here are of use to you, please use them with yourself and with your patients. If they do not seem useful, let them go; no need to worry about them further. We wish well-being, wisdom, loving-kindness, and freedom from suffering for you and your patients.

The Foundational Elements of Buddhist Psychology
The Four "Noble Truths"

Life is full of misery, loneliness, and suffering—and it's all over much too soon.

—WOODY ALLEN

By now, most CBT practitioners have noticed the aforementioned flood of mindfulness- and acceptance-based methods that have strongly affected our field. These methods have typically been added to our therapy toolbox as a part of a packaged mode of practice, such as DBT (Linehan, 1993a) or MBSR (Kabat Zinn, 1990). While useful, these mindfulness-, acceptance-, and compassion-informed psychotherapies present concepts derived from Buddhist psychology as separate from the philosophical context from which they have emerged. So if one wishes to move beyond this trend of importing mindfulness techniques into psychotherapy, and move toward a true integration of Buddhist psychology and CBT, this path will involve an understanding of the most fundamental principles of the philosophy of the Buddhism.

DHARMA

"Buddhism" is a 19th-century Western term for the psychological methodology attributed to the historical teacher known as the Buddha. This set of practices was originally known as *dharma*, which can be translated as "way," "law," or "sacred duty." In Buddhism, *dharma* most commonly refers to the body of Buddhist teachings. However, the term can be found in nearly all of the philosophical and wellness-based systems that have emerged from the Indian subcontinent (Kalupahana, 1986). Looking at the range of such philosophies as a whole, a more universal definition of *dharma* emerges that stands for the natural laws of the universe (Mosig, 1989; Thurman, 1997). These laws were said to provide for order, harmony, and life by creating cycles of interacting processes (Kwee, 2011). While it may seem like a mystical assumption to assume that a universal law holds all reality together, our own science establishes just such premises. When we think of axiomatic scientific terms, such as "gravity," "energy," or even "cognition," we encounter the culturally perceived universal laws of our era. Similarly the "laws" of mathematics or physics, or the principles of evolution and behavior, are all considered to reflect the way our world organizes itself and behaves.

Hence, *dharma* links the Buddha's teachings with the established understanding of the observable universe during the time of the Buddha's life. Similarly, many cognitive and behavioral therapies seek to situate their philosophy and approach in evolutionary science, affective neuroscience, and experimental psychology of behavior (Atkinson & Wheeler, 2003). Like the Buddha, cognitive and behavioral practitioners have connected our laws and working concepts to what we know about how life emerges on the planet, and how organisms behave in context (Hofmann, 2012). So as the the *dharma* of Buddhism and the *dharma* of CBT evolve into one another, we turn to the basic architecture: the first and perhaps most important teachings of the the Buddha: the "Four Noble Truths" and the "Noble Eightfold Path."

THE STORY OF THE HISTORICAL BUDDHA AND THE FOUR NOBLE TRUTHS

When Westerners first learn about Buddhism, they often discover the biography of the venerated historical teacher Siddartha Gotama, who became known as "the one who woke up" or the *Buddha*. Indeed, the mythologized tale of the founder of Buddhism is a fundamental teaching tool in Buddhist psychology. As we will see, the life story of the historical Buddha leads us directly to an understanding of his foundational teaching, known as the *Four Noble Truths*. Interestingly, when we consider the story of the historical Buddha, we may find that we have much in common with him. While the cultural and technological worlds that surround us and the Buddha may be dissimilar, today's CBT therapists and Siddartha Gotama share a common motivation and a common course of action in their lives. Both the therapist and the Buddha have been so moved by the suffering that they have witnessed around them, they have dedicated their lives to better understand how the mind works and how they might free their fellow human beings from suffering through the application of rationality, wisdom, and deep personal inquiry. So, whether or not you realized your common purpose with the Buddha when you woke up this morning, you can rest your head on your pillow tonight, remembering that you are in highly regarded company in your life's mission.

As history and legend have told us, Siddartha Gotama was born on the Indian subcontinent, as a prince of a region in what is now known as Nepal, approximately 2,600 years ago. According to historical records and myths, it was prophesied that this prince would either rise to power as a great king, or would pursue a life of spiritual practice, eventually leading to a spiritual awakening. According to the mythopoetic accounts of Siddartha Gotama's life, his father had a desire for his son to enter the "family business," living life as a monarch rather than as a monastic. It is taught that his father took great effort to surround him with finery and luxury, filling his life with pleasure, and shielding him from the unpleasantness and suffering of the world around him, in the hope that this would steer Siddartha toward a life of temporal power rather than a pursuit of personal enlightenment (Goldstein & Kornfield, 1987). Famously, Siddartha eventually saw past his life of luxury when he was confronted with the more tragic aspects of life, but his myth tells us that his youth was spent endlessly engaged in pleasurable pursuits, athletic games, and absorption in the enjoyment of a wealthy life of leisure.

Very few of us are royalty, or live with boundless privilege. However, if we consider our lives in contrast to the environment in which Siddartha lived, the Himalayas in the sixth century B.C.E., we will likely find that we live in luxury. Siddartha didn't live in an era of indoor plumbing, central air conditioning, or antibiotics, let alone iPads and air travel. Indeed, those of us in the 21st-century "developed world" need only to pause and remember that 80% of the current human population lives on less than ten dollars per day, in order to realize the extent of our truly good fortune (Chen & Ravallion, 2008).

Just as Siddartha Gotama's father sought to surround his son with distracting luxury and pleasure, we too may have filled our lives with items and conditions designed to shield us from the pain, misery, and uncertainty of the world around us, such as big-screen televisions with hundreds of channels, and websites that transmit our entertainment of choice 24 hours a day. For many, the pursuit of pleasure and distraction may also involve indulgence in food, alcohol, sex, and recreational drugs. And just as Siddartha did, we may find that these distractions are inadequate when we are confronted with the harsher realities of life. We may sense a disquiet that there is something lying behind the curtain of the good times. Perhaps we sense that no degree of sensory pleasure can erase the inevitable pain and uncertainty of life, or bring us lasting satisfaction and happiness. As the Buddha did, we may have sensed that the secrets to obtaining happiness and peace cannot be bought, but must be discovered and cultivated. Like him, we may find ourselves stepping out into the world, only to discover the harder edges of the human experience.

The original tales of the life of Siddartha tell us that he eventually traveled outside the walls of his palace, only to witness the human suffering that everyday people were experiencing all around him in his sheltered world. In this way, he discovered a basic truth that many of us are confronted with daily, in our own lives and in the lives of our patients. Siddartha discovered suffering as he witnessed his fellow human beings encounter old age, sickness, and death. The pain of others touched him, and he experienced pain himself. This fundamental act of empathy and perspective taking brought about a great motivation to help alleviate the suffering he encountered in the world. As we will see, such a capacity for empathy and seeing life through the eyes of others is an important part of the adaptive psychological processes pursued in CBT and Buddhist psychology.

As many of us who have chosen to go into the helping professions have experienced, Siddartha found himself deeply, emotionally moved in the face of human suffering, and committed his life to understanding it, and to freeing himself and others from suffering. In the 21st century, earnest young people in the developed world who are seeking to alleviate psychological suffering might go to graduate school or medical school. For the man who became known as the Buddha, the path to wisdom and liberation from suffering led to living and training with ascetics and monks who had renounced material pleasures, and devoted themselves to contemplative practices and bodily disciplines.

As part of an oral tradition, the mystics and wandering sages of the Himalayas and the Indian subcontinent served as living repositories of centuries-old methods for training the mind and the body. Their methods would probably seem remarkably austere, even masochistic, to most of the readers of this book; they practiced things like abstaining from food and denying themselves physical pleasures of any kind. However, these were the practitioners of wisdom and emotional healing that existed in Siddartha's context, and this is where his aim to alleviate human suffering took him. Siddartha left the comfort and security of his home and family to pursue the personal transformation he believed would lead to unlocking the secret of the alleviation of human suffering.

After years of practicing the most austere ascetic disciplines, the man who became known as the Buddha came to believe that abasement of the flesh and self-abnegation were neither necessary nor sufficient conditions for liberation from suffering. He came to engage deeply with meditative disciplines that involved silently and nonjudgmentally witnessing the ebb and flow of his conscious mind, espousing what he described as a "Middle Path" that did not involve self-inflicted punishment, but that moved the practitioner toward an experience of compassion, willingness, wisdom, and a transcendent experience of selfhood, that he believed could transform the mind and lead to a complete liberation from suffering and an elevation of consciousness. As the mythopoetic history of the Buddha is told, the Buddha sat beneath a tree, in a state of deep meditation, resolving to remain there until he became a fully realized being, enlightened to the nature of all things, transcending suffering. As he sat, many projections of his mind, worries, ambitions, and concerns arose in his awareness, just as many distractions may flow through the mind of the novice meditator. However, the Buddha remained in his meditative state of awareness through the rising and falling away of all of these experiences, until a clear seeing and a transcendent sense of self emerged.

The story of the Buddha achieving realization and deep personal awakening to the true nature of self, reality, and the phenomenal realm, which is to say, of his enlightenment, is well known. We all likely can conjure an image of the Indian sage sitting beneath the Bodhi tree, in a state of peaceful joyfulness. This image, of course, is a solitary one, and it does not immediately suggest an engagement with the rest of the world, carrying this wisdom forward to help alleviate the suffering of others. In fact, traditional tales of the Buddha tell us that he was, at first, reluctant to teach or disseminate his observations or methods. In time, the historical Buddha did come to share his observations and his techniques with students. Remarkably, the Buddha's methods are available to us today, as is thousands of years of empirical evidence supporting these practices, in the form of the teachings of countless meditators, Buddhist practitioners, and monks, who have followed the systematic program put forward by the Buddha for the alleviation of suffering. As we will see, the current state of psychological outcome, process, and neuroimaging research corroborates the insights and technologies developed by the Buddha.

In order to understand the Buddha's method, we begin with his fundamental teaching, that of the Four Noble Truths. These truths serve as a point of view, a place to stand, a series of fundamental assumptions from which the entirety of Buddhist psychology can be seen to emerge. CBT literature does not usually use terms that are as lofty as "noble" and "truth" to describe its theory and methods. In fact, part of the reason Buddhist psychology contains language that sounds so ecumenical and grand is that the initial translators of the texts of the *dharma* in the West tended to be Christian scholars, who were looking to establish correspondences across the world's religions. When we look at these Four Noble Truths, we are actually looking at one of the earliest psychological accounts of the fundamental processes involved in human suffering, and the first method of addressing suffering that has its roots in a theory of mind based on observation of reality rather than religious assumptions. In fact, the theoretical assumptions of the Four Noble Truths are very much in accord with CBT concepts, which may explain why there is so much room for technical integration between Buddhist psychology and CBT.

Soothing Rhythm Breathing

Before beginning our exploration of the Four Noble Truths, it is useful to ground ourselves in practice, beginning with bringing our attention to the rhythm of our breath. Meditation in Buddhist traditions pervades so much of the experience and path that practitioners follow. The states of mind and body that meditation cultivates are not meant to be rarified experiences that are only available during religious rituals. In fact, the qualities of mind that are trained in Buddhist psychology are meant to become lasting attributes of a person's everyday being and behavior.

The practice below is adapted from the foundational breathing meditation found in CFT (Gilbert, 2010a), described as the "soothing rhythm breathing." Our practice is derived from elements of both Buddhist concentration and mindfulness meditation, and is adapted into a brief and clearly understandable form, usable in the context of psychotherapy. As such, it serves as an apt illustration of the integration of Buddhist psychology and CBT, from the ground up. The meditation invites us to find a point of stillness in our experience of breathing, from which we may observe the comings and goings of our mind. This stillness involves the activation of the parasympathetic nervous system, calming, and relaxation, which all involve "coherent breathing" (Brown & Gerbarg, 2012). Similar practices are a part of "classical mindfulness" (Rapgay & Bystrisky, 2009), Tibetan *shamatha* meditation, and Zen meditation.

When practiced as an element of CFT, soothing rhythm breathing is used with a range of clients who present with a variety of psychological difficulties. As such, therapists who are beginning their work with clients seeking treatment for anxiety or mood disorders, and who wish to move on to subsequent mindfulness, acceptance, and compassion-based practice, may find it useful to train clients in the basics of soothing rbythm breathing during the earlier sessions of therapy. From this foundation, a variety of more advanced practices can be developed.

For the following rhythmic breathing practice, use the directions provided to help guide and structure the practice, all the while allowing your experience to lead you, using your own words and pacing. This exercise is usually conducted in a seated position with the back straight, yet supple. The ideal setting should be comfortable and in a place and time where you will be free from distraction or interruption:

Guided Instructions

As we will often begin our practices, please find a comfortable place to be, where you can place both of your feet on the floor, and can allow your back to adopt a straight and supple posture. As much as you can, allow yourself to feel settled and grounded into the experience. When you feel willing, allow your eyes to close, perhaps adopting a friendly or relaxed facial expression, perhaps smiling slightly. Begin to draw your attention to the gentle flow of the breath in and out of the body. Feel your connection to the breath as you inhale and exhale. As best you can, hold your focus on the breath with a gentle and allowing spirit, not aiming to change or correct anything at all, but simply being with the act of breathing.

As you begin to deepen your awareness of the flow of the breath, feel your breath descend into the belly, noticing the rise and fall of the abdomen and chest. As best you can, allow the air to reach the bottom of your lungs. As you exhale, notice the falling or gentle shrinking of the abdomen. Feel the muscles under the ribcage moving with each inhale. As you notice the rising and falling of the belly, allow your breath to find its own rhythm and its own pace, simply allowing the breath to breathe itself, just giving way to your breath's own rhythm, moment by moment. With each in-breath, feel as if you are breathing attention into the body, and with each out-breath, let go.

Now, extending and lengthening the outbreath, allow the breath to settle into a slow, soothing rhythm. Breathing in, count for 3 seconds, pause for a moment, now release the out-breath for 3 seconds. As you, can, extend this rhythm to 4 seconds of in-breath and out-breath, and then to 5 seconds. Hold this timing lightly, using it as a guide and a pulse. Whenever your mind wanders away to thoughts, images, or distractions, gently remember that this is the nature of mind. Upon the next in-breath, bring your attention back to this soothing rhythm of the breath.

Remain with this attention to the soothing rhythm of your breath as long as you can, feeling the breath descending through the lungs, noticing the rising and falling of the abdomen, and sensing the release of the exhalation.

After practicing this soothing rhythm breathing for a few minutes, allow yourself to notice when you are ready to bring this practice to a close. Then, exhale and to let go of this exercise entirely. At your own pace, bring your awareness back into your surroundings and open your eyes, returning to your experience right now.

Based on exercises in Gilbert (2010a); and adapted from Tirch (2012). Reprinted with permission from New Harbinger Publications, Inc., and Little, Brown Book Group. Copyright 2012 by Dennis Tirch.

The First Noble Truth: Dukkha

The First Noble Truth sets out the problem that the Buddha sought to solve. It is *dukkha*, a Pali (archaic Sanskrit) word that is often translated to mean "suffering." The First Noble Truth suggests that every aspect of life will involve some element of dissatisfaction, some imbalance, and some degree of pain. While a translation of *dukkha* as "suffering" isn't exactly incorrect, it is incomplete (Rahula, 1959/1974). The root of the word represents the feeling of riding in a wagon, when one of the wheels is out of balance. The problem with translating *dukkha* as "suffering" is that it is often taken to mean that the Buddha taught that all of life is nothing but pain and suffering. What a depressing approach to life, let alone psychological healing! In fact, when the Tibetan Buddhist nun and writer Thubten Chodron was consulted by one of us (R. L. K.), she was quick to suggest, "Whatever you do, don't tell them Buddhists just think that life is suffering!"

We suspect Thubten Chodron isn't the only Buddhist who has found herself all too aware of this misinterpretation of the Buddha's First Noble Truth. This idea has likely caused thousands to believe that the Buddhist approach to life is pessimistic. It's easy to see how these sorts of misconceptions arise, however, because even some Buddhist teachers seem to communicate exactly this lesson of suffering. If this were the first thing we learned about the Buddha's teaching, we could perhaps be excused for shaking our heads and moving on to something that isn't quite so depressing.

A complete definition of *dukkha* is much more expansive, and would include descriptors such as "imperfect," "impermanent," "frustrating," and perhaps "fundamentally and ultimately unsatisfying" (Das, 1997; Rahula, 1959/1974). And while the First Noble Truth does focus on suffering (in the way that much of psychology has historically focused on suffering—because that is what is being addressed), the Buddha also taught in numerous places the importance of finding happiness (Nhat Hahn, 1998).

The essence of the First Noble Truth is that life is difficult, and in several different ways. The Buddha described three types of *dukkha* (Rahula, 1959/1974). First, there's the suffering that comes with having a human life: we all age, get sick, and die. We all lose people we love, and most of us will have our hearts broken, sustain injuries, do our best and fail, be ridiculed or insulted, and experience countless other experiences of pain, difficulty, inconvenience, or disappointment during our lives. Our lives are short, perhaps 25,000 to 30,000 days if we are lucky. Our bodies are prone to all sorts of diseases and injuries. The satisfaction we take in the pleasure and pride of the physical body is subject to the inevitable decline of aging. All of this contributes to *dukkha-dukkha*, which we will call "the basic suffering of living." Again, this isn't to say that *all* of life is suffering. It simply means that a certain amount of pain and difficulty comes with having a human life and a physical body—it's unavoidable—and coming to terms with this reality is important.

The second type of *dukkha* is *viparinama-dukkha*, which we will call "the suffering of change." We pursue pleasure and happiness in any number of ways, but what happens when we've gotten what we want? Eventually, things change. We're happy with our jobs, and then a new CEO or dean is hired who changes everything around. The perfect evening ends; the heat of a new relationship fades; our stylish jacket becomes a sign that we're hopelessly stuck in the 1990s. We know this phenomenon happens not only in the world, as a result of changing circumstances, but in our minds as well. Our minds become excited by novelty but then habituate, our excitement fading even if the stimulus that caused it remains unchanged. Just when we think we've got everything we need to be happy, the game changes and we find ourselves on the hunt again.

The third, most profound, and elusive form of *dukkha* is *samkhara-dukkha*, which refers to the ephemeral nature of existence. We will call this "the suffering of conditioned reality." This form of *dukkha* is perhaps the most difficult for a mind trained in the Western tradition to grasp, and is also most core to the philosophical basis of the Buddhist understanding of reality. At its most basic level, we can consider this form of suffering as a result of the fact that things decay—that nothing has permanent, unchanging existence—and that ultimately all things will pass into other forms of existence (Nhat Hanh, 1998). From a certain point of view, absolutely everything—from the level of subatomic particles up to the most complex forms of life, even systems of planets and stars—is actively involved in a process of falling apart, transforming into something else, and ultimately ceasing to exist in its current state.

Clinical Example

The following clinical example illustrates how an appreciation of the universality of human suffering can help to guide a Buddhist psychology-informed CBT intervention. It describes an interaction with a CBT practitioner and a client who is being treated for posttraumatic stress disorder (PTSD). Our client, Rita, is a 35-year-old woman with a history of repeated childhood medical trauma. As a result of her PTSD experience, a range of human relationships, career tasks, and other environmental challenges can trigger painful and seemingly overwhelming emotional memories, as well as flashbacks. In a recent session, Rita and her therapist discussed how the fluorescent lights in the therapist's waiting room triggered emotional reexperiencing of threat emotions related to her medical traumas. Although the compassion-focused cognitive restructuring intervention that they worked with was reportedly helpful, Rita felt great shame after her session was over. Dutifully completing homework to question her automatic thoughts concerning her present-moment safety, she still felt shame that she had experienced and discussed flashbacks at all. The therapist and the client discussed Rita's experiences in the light of the First Noble Truth. This wasn't done in an explicitly Buddhist way, but by using Socratic questioning drawn from cognitive therapy and CFT, emotional self-disclosure from FAP and

ACT, and the basic human empathic connection that all psychotherapies share as we turn toward the suffering of ourselves and the world.

CLIENT: Last week when we talked about how anxious and triggered I was by the lights in the office, I just felt so humiliated afterward. It's hard to even talk about. *(Looks tearful and afraid.)*

THERAPIST: I'm encouraged that you want to go a bit further in working with that today, Rita. I can see that you look sad, and even a bit scared. Last session, talking about being triggered felt very important. It was very brave of you.

CLIENT: *(smiling, while crying softly)* Thanks for telling me that. I really appreciated that you helped me to learn to do something when I was triggered. We didn't just explore the feeling, and we didn't run away from it. I used the new responding homework all week. It's just that . . . after we talked about it, I felt so pathetic. Like, I can't even sit in my doctor's office without feeling threatened. I'm so ashamed.

THERAPIST: Shame can show up so quickly and so naturally for us, even if there isn't anything we could have done. This sounds very heavy for you to carry today.

CLIENT: It is, but I deserve it. I'm so weak and pathetic.

THERAPIST: Can I ask you a few questions about this experience?

CLIENT: Yes, of course.

THERAPIST: Rita, did you choose to be born in this part of the world at this period of time? *(Smiles.)*

CLIENT: *(gently laughing)* No. That's impossible.

THERAPIST: And did you choose your parents, or your physical body, which, like all of ours, is prone to problems?

CLIENT: Of course not. I didn't ask for any of this.

THERAPIST: That's right, isn't it? Wow! You didn't ask for any of this. None of us asks for this. We are born with tricky brains and bodies that can have such problems. We age, and we get sick. Eventually we even die. And we don't choose our parents, our schools, or our classmates. So much in life is not what we would choose and is really not our fault.

CLIENT: No, it really isn't. I'm so angry that I had all of that happen to me. I'm so sad and so angry, and it is just awful.

THERAPIST: It really is sad that you have had these painful events in your life. It is sad and it makes me angry that you have had to suffer this way. I want you to know that it really is just not your fault. There is nothing broken in us when we feel emotional pain and deal with difficult, difficult things in life. We all feel shame in some way. We all feel pain. Your pain, here and now, pains me. And we can know that you did not ask for it. We can know that this is not your fault.

CLIENT: *(pausing for a long time)* I know I'm not alone, you know? It is going to take some time to work on these things. I get that it's not my fault. It won't just go away, but it helps to know that this is a part of life for everyone, one way or another. Ugh. It really sucks though. *(Smiles.)*

This first vignette illustrates the kind of encounter that the First Noble Truth suggests. We begin where we are, with gentle, compassionate acceptance of our shared suffering. Unlike many clinical examples in many texts, this example does not end with the problems solved. Because so few exchanges in life do, in fact, end in that way. We approach our work to transform our suffering into possibility with mindfulness, courage, and compassion. We approach our clients suffering with as much openness and wisdom as we can bring to this present moment. And, in this way, our work begins in Buddhist psychology-informed CBT.

Conditioned Reality, Self, and Suffering

Looking more closely, "the suffering of conditioned reality" (*samkhara-dukkha*) gives us a window into the Buddhist understanding of the nature of reality itself. From the perspective of the *dharma*, as in some schools of physics, all things are intimately interconnected, and have their foundations in infinitesimal fluctuations of the very stuff of space–time. In this point of view, any perceived separateness is ultimately an illusion, and exists in the mind of the perceiver. Concepts this abstract may not have immediately apparent relevance to the practical work of the CBT therapist. However, assumptions based on these concepts can significantly inform our interventions.

In the world of psychology, we spend a good deal of time discussing, researching, hypothesizing about, and developing treatments that both rely on and are designed to address psychological constructs. These constructs—things like "depression," "cognitive schemas," "attachment bonds," and "self-esteem"—are both interesting and tricky. On the one hand, we talk about them almost as things in themselves, reifying constructs into objects. We seek to develop, maneuver, or change these ideas; we may even (perhaps mistakenly) refer to them as causal agents. But we also know that these things don't really exist as separate, physical entities unto themselves. We can't locate them, point to them, or measure them purely and directly. All of these constructs are language-based descriptions of the experiences and behaviors of human beings in context. None exist in and of themselves.

We infer these constructs, because they have explanatory power: they help us to label and efficiently communicate our experience to others. Psychological constructs serve to capture some aspect of cognition, emotion, or experience. They also help us to connect the dots between hypothesized causes and effects—like explaining how an abusive childhood history may lead to an adult who finds it difficult to function in relationships. Like physicists including dark matter into our equations because the equations just don't work if we don't, we rely upon these constructs as we attempt to understand and explain human behavior, and aim to alleviate suffering. But we know these things have no inherent reality. They exist, predominantly, in our minds.

For example, we *seem* to know "love" when we see it, but in practice love as an emotion or action is difficult to define or observe in the moment. This is precisely why psychologists spend so much time designing and publishing assessment instruments: because many of the things we are interested in can't be measured directly. They are insubstantial, they are ephemeral, and their reality is inferred rather than known. The Buddhist characterization of our experience as including the suffering of conditioned reality reminds us that the impermanent and insubstantial nature of these constructs can be unsettling when we stop to consider them. In a sense, our psychological concepts give us nothing to grab onto, and as we'll see with the Second Noble Truth, we very much want to have something to hold onto, to find a sense of certainty and stability.

Our discomfort with the limits of our experiencing can be a powerful motivator—spawning, for example, the behavioral revolution in psychology, as our field sought to optimally predict and influence human behavior with precision, depth, and scope, without resorting to reification of mentalistic explanatory constructs (Fletcher, Schoendorff, & Hayes, 2010; Hayes, Luoma, Bond, Masuda, & Lillis, 2006). This behavioral revolution led to many of the most effective methods for alleviating human psychological suffering. However, even at the edges of an attempt to forgo the use of psychological constructs, we find our limits. For the behaviorist, all mental events exist in a context, and are essentially dependent variables. So, automatic thoughts are not the cause of our suffering, but are viewed as internal behaviors that we engage in as a response to our context. All of our words, even the words of behaviorism itself, are ultimately symbols, and depend upon a human mind for their relevance and meaning.

So, the suffering of conditioned reality (*samkhara-dukkha*) posits that every individual aspect of the greater totality of the universe is absent of inherent existence (Malalasekera, 1966). All phenomena are so interdependent and interconnected that any slicing or division of the observable world into separate parts has no intrinsic reality, even if it may have practical utility. Particularly when applied to the self, this concept of the absence of inherent existence presents us with questions that can be disquieting to consider and seemingly impossible to answer: "Who am I?", "What can be counted on?", "What is the self, and how can I know it?"

We use the word "I" countless times during the course of even a single day, but what does it mean, really? "Who am 'I?'"; "What am 'I?'"; and "Where am 'I' to be found?" From the Buddhist perspective, there is no concrete "self" that can be found. Rather, the self is seen as a construct that is inferred from the observation of the ever-changing flow of physical and mental processes, described in terms of five primary constituents: matter, sensation, perceptions, mental formations, and consciousness (Rahula, 1959/1974). These constituents themselves, in turn, lack substantiality and separateness.

Buddhist psychology suggests that we can't observe the self directly. We observe our act of thinking, and we infer the presence of a self. This conception shares a great deal of common ground with the core concept of the self from a behavioral analytic perspective, wherein the experience of a self emerges from our responding to our own responding (Stewart, Villatte, & McHugh, 2012). From a Buddhist perspective, even thinking itself is considered to have no inherent existence. This is what Buddhists would call "conditioned existence," within which the self exists entirely in dependence upon the causes and conditions that produce it, and without those conditions it would not exist. Even the use of the term "conditioned" reveals a philosophical resonance between

Buddhism and behaviorism: both view the interaction of changes in context as the conditions that bring forth our apparent experience of being. B. F. Skinner (1974) himself might have appreciated this Buddhist self-formulation, as he has written: "A person is not an originating agent. He is a locus, a point at which many genetic and environmental conditions come together in a joint effect" (p. 168).

Buddhist psychology applies a similar logic to our experience of what we call "reality," ultimately reducing our moment-to-moment experience to mental "snapshots" that seem to solidify what is actually a constantly changing interplay of causes, conditions, forces, and energies. Things come together to shape what we experience in this moment, and later, they decay and come apart again, becoming something different in an ever-flowing chain of causes and conditions.

Those of us with even the most basic background in behavior analysis or dialectical behavior therapy may find this line of thinking familiar when we recall the concept of behavioral "chains" or "behavioral chain analysis" (Linehan, 1993a). When we seek to understand a behavior, we often can't comprehend it in isolation. We need to consider the causes and conditions that maintain it—the antecedents that signal its occurrence, and the consequences that maintain it. If we look at a certain behavior such as nonsuicidal self-injury or "cutting," it may at first seem quite difficult to understand. It is only when we consider the causes and conditions that produced the behavior (extreme emotional pain) and the consequences that reinforce it (the reduction of that pain), that we can truly understand what we are seeing.

From the Buddhist psychology perspective, the cutting does not, and cannot, exist independently of the pain and the motivation to alleviate it, just as the relief of pain does not exist independent of its causes (in this example, the cutting). As we become practiced at considering causes and conditions, we can begin to see human lives as ongoing sequences of behaviors and experiences, in which each behavior or experience serves as a consequence of those that preceded it, and the antecedent to the next behavior or experience in line. Of course, our behaviors and experiences are acted upon by many other factors, including the genetic variations in affective responding, cognitive processes, the actions of other beings, different occurrences in our environments, and the external outcomes that follow our actions. Over time, our behaviors and interactions take on patterns, which we observe, become familiar with, and organize in our minds into mental formations—ideas and schemas that we then relate to as "I"—an "I" which, from the Buddhist perspective, is impermanent, transitory, and entirely dependent upon the causes and conditions that shaped it.

Ultimately, the First Noble Truth isn't so much a message of dire consequence as it is one of acceptance of the fundamental nature of our apparent reality as it dynamically presents itself to us, moment by moment. In a culture that all too often may seem to communicate that we should always be happy and should never suffer, and equipped as we are with brains and bodies that naturally and reflexively recoil from pain, the Buddha tells us that pain and suffering are a simple fact of life—if we are to be alive, we're going to face them (sickness, pain, loss, death). The irony of it is that the more we seem to avoid this reality, the more suffering we bring upon ourselves.

This perspective is hardly a new one to the cognitive-behavior therapist. Numerous therapeutic traditions have acknowledged the significant role of attempting to avoid painful experiences and emotions in the etiology of a wide variety of psychological disturbances and maladaptive behaviors including substance abuse, trauma response, and anxiety disorders more broadly (Chawla & Ostafin, 2007; Salters-Pedneault, Tull, & Roemer, 2004). Additionally, experiential avoidance has been proposed as a fundamental transdiagnostic dimension hypothesized to underlie numerous behavioral disturbances (Hayes, Wilson, Gifford, Follette, & Strosahl, 1996), a theoretical perspective that lies at the very heart of ACT (Hayes, Strosahl, & Wilson, 2011). Much of what has arisen during the third wave of CBT has involved an acceptance of suffering, a suspension of attachment to our mental constructs, and the generation and extension of self-compassion. All of these ideas have their antecedents in Buddhist psychology.

The Flow of Life of Meditation

Meditative healing traditions have been using the imagination to facilitate emotionally positive experiences for centuries before the birth of the historical Buddha. Notably, Tibetan lineages and some Japanese lineages use visualization to guide the mind and to stimulate certain mental experiences. We know that imaginary events can stimulate the same regions of the brain, and even evoke the same behaviors, as events in the world (Dymond, Roche, & Bennett, 2013). For example, if I am hungry and imagine my favorite food, I'm very likely to salivate and my stomach will secrete digestive fluids. Use this exercise as an introduction to how imagery can guide the mind and stimulate the brain. Furthermore, see if you can use the experience of this practice to contact the felt sense of intercon-nectedness that Buddhist psychology describes in its theoretical writings.

This exercise can be used to illustrate our place in the evolutionary flow of life on the planet. This teaching point can be used to help cultivate self-compas-sion, as we realize how much that we experience in life is not of our choosing, and is not our fault. This practice is compatible with many of the third-generation CBT protocols that use imagery, or that seek to train clients in a flexible sense of self. Clients who begin therapy with dissociative symptoms and a trauma history might not be the best candidates for deeper or prolonged use of imag-ery, particularly early in therapy. Nevertheless, many clients who are engaged in a process of developing mindfulness, compassion, and imagery-building skills might benefit from this practice, and its experiential illustration of our emerging, interconnected, and flexible self-experiences.

Guided Instructions

Finding a comfortable and quiet place to sit, begin by simply noticing the physi-cal sensations that present themselves to you, here and now. Closing your eyes, notice the sounds that are around you. Observe the feeling of your feet on the floor, your weight in your chair, and your back, straight and supported. Bringing your attention to the flow of your breath, gather your attention and engage your soothing rhythm breathing. Take a minute or two to follow the breath, finding a grounded stillness in your posture, and in the even flow of your breath. Whenever your mind wanders, make space for that experience, and return to the present moment, with accepting and kind awareness, by following the in-breath. Take this moment outside of clock time to rest in kindness, and to rest in the flow of your breath.

Now we will begin forming an image in the mind. However this image emerges, in whatever clarity or however shifting, that is perfectly okay. You are okay just as you are, in this very moment. Imagine that you are standing before the vastness of the ocean, with your feet on a sandy beach. In your mind, you are watching the clear blue color of the water, and noticing the waves softly land against the sand and rocks. Watching the rolling waves, you notice the point in the distance where the sky meets the water. Hold this image lightly, it may change or vary, and as much as you can see if you can picture yourself stand-ing at the shore, in the shallow water of the beach. Feel the warm water gently engulfing your feet and ankles. Imagine that you can notice the sand between your toes and underneath the soles of your feet as the water moves up and down the shore. Feel the breeze as it cools your skin and body that has been warmed by the sun. See the brightness of the sunlight as it reflects off the water, using all of your senses to create this experience in the mind. Imagine that you can smell the fresh air from the sea, and feel this air moving through you.

Bring your awareness to the horizon, noticing the vastness of the ocean, an ocean that has been in existence for countless thousands of years. All life on our planet begins in the water, and, in a sense, in this very ocean before you. The ocean has been witness to the many periods of change on this planet: the birth and death of millions of species of life, the rise and fall of the earth's climates, the shifting of the tectonic plates and formation of mountains, rivers, forests, deserts, and glaciers. Over a period of time that is more expansive than we can even comprehend, this water has moved, giving birth to the flow of life on our Earth, and giving birth to us. We have come out of the world, not into it. We have emerged from this flow of life, from this ancient living presence. Now, as best you can, see if you can imagine that this old and vast ocean completely accepts you, just as you are, here and now. This ocean knows your history, knows your struggles, and knows your suffering, and sees you as significant beloved being in an interconnected flow of life. This wise and ancient ocean, the source of all of who we are, knows that you are awake, alert, and alive. You are a mindful being connected to the on-goingness of everything around you. In this moment, allow yourself to feel connected to this ocean, to its silent wisdom, to its power, and to its acceptance. Recognizing that we are all a part of the evolution of life on this shared planet, intimately, and physically connected to all that surrounds us, allow yourself to rest in the wisdom of this present moment. When you are ready, let this image go and bring your attention back to your presence in the chair, and in the room. With a deep exhalation, let the entire exercise go, and bring your attention back to here and now, reengaging with your day.

Based on an exercise in Gilbert (2009a).

The Second Noble Truth: The Origin of Suffering

The Second Noble Truth relates to how our suffering, dissatisfaction, and frustrations come to arise. In considering these issues, we might see the Buddha as a master psychologist. From the Buddha's perspective, it wasn't the pain of life, the fact that things change, or even that everything is impermanent and decays that causes our suffering. The content and the substrate of life itself does not produce suffering, according to the perspective of the Buddha. Our response to these events, to these conditions, is the primary proximal cause of our ongoing state of suffering, according to the Second Noble Truth. Buddhist psychology describes this source of our suffering as *tanha*, which literally means "thirst." We can think of *tanha* as a powerful and never-ending experience of thirst, craving, or clinging attachment (Das, 1997; Rahula, 1959/1974). According to the Second Noble Truth, our suffering is caused by craving or thirsting for those things we don't have (or feel we don't have enough of), and by struggling to avoid or push away those things we don't wish to have. We suffer to the degree that we are unable or unwilling to accept the present moment as it is, with willingness, equanimity, and ease.

Our natural evolutionarily necessary response to our environment involves moving away from those events in our environment that we deem as aversive, and moving toward what appears appetitive (Ramnero

& Torneke, 2008). This is part of the most basic dynamics of being alive. However, the human animal, with its remarkably complex mental capacities, is capable of great desires and the mental construction of a myriad of hypothetical situations in which we are happier, healthier, or experiencing greater pleasure. As such, we are easily captured by powerful cravings for things that we want, and the variations in things that we can crave are almost endless. We thirst for material possessions: money, property, luxuries, and other sense pleasures.

We crave relationships, respect, power, and status. These powerful desires and tendencies to cling even apply to ideas, perspectives, opinions, and theories. As we will see in our discussion of the various emotion regulation systems that are present in the human brain, mind, and body, recent advances in affective neuroscience have isolated a particular motivational system that involves seeking out resources, pleasure, and achieving goals (Pani, Porcella, & Gessa, 2000; Panksepp, 1998). This acquisition-based system, involving the neurotransmitter dopamine in particular, is a powerful evolutionary tool for pursuing what sustains us as a species. However, as individuals, we may vary in the degree to which this emotional system dominates and influences our behavior. The Second Noble Truth suggests that an overemphasis on craving and desire leads to a struggle with the experience of things as they are, and an increase in the experience of *dukkha*.

Our evolved attachment to the pursuit of goals can lead us to become locked in what is referred to in Buddhist psychology as "neurotic craving" even when the object of our craving is abstract. Under such conditions, we can become overidentified with ideas and tribal identifications, and lose sight of responsiveness to the present moment and to a sense of our common humanity. It's easy to point at politicians for examples of emotional outbursts based on ideological differences, but one can find plenty of examples at psychology conferences as well. Haven't we all been occasionally taken aback by heated exchanges in public forums by otherwise civilized psychologists over what seem to be minor theoretical differences? We all feel the pull of craving, attachment, and desire, and even those who seek to remedy this problem can find themselves in its thrall. Religious wars are another example where one side is pitted against the other, both ready to murder one another in massive numbers so that their version of peace, love, and understanding will be supreme. All of this is a bit of oversimplification, but it is important to recognize the ubiquity of the implications of this Second Noble Truth.

The Origin of Suffering, Learning Theory, and Experiential Avoidance

On the one hand, our behavioral repertoires can be dominated by neurotic craving and an overzealous experience of being driven by desire. On the other hand, we find the second dominating source of *dukkha*, of human suffering, is the powerful influence of aversion. We not only experience strong desires to pursue and then cling to the things we want, but we can also experience powerful negative reactions when faced with situations, experiences, or ideas that we don't like.

This perspective is certainly consistent with a variety of theories within the CBT family. Beginning with basic learning theory, we find that the cores of both classical and operant conditioning are based in our powerful tendencies to pursue some outcomes and avoid others. Whether we are learning on the basis of associating stimuli in our environment (classical conditioning), or learning through the consequences of our actions (operant conditioning), much of what we learn is driven by the experiences of pleasure and displeasure, desire and aversion (Domjan, 1998; Zajonc, 1984).

Our brains form powerful classically conditioned associations between those environmental events that produce desirable or undesirable emotional (or physical) experiences and the previously neutral stimuli that seem to signal these events (Ramnero & Torneke, 2008). The tendency to pursue some outcomes and avoid others provides the foundation for operant learning too,, as we predictably repeat behaviors that lead to favorable outcomes (or, in the case of negative reinforcement, terminate undesirable experiences or situations), and attempt to refrain from behaviors that do not produce such outcomes (or that produce the opposite outcome). In conducting a functional analysis of behavior, in which we closely examine the factors that signal the onset of a behavior and those behaviors that maintain it, we are in a sense exploring the dynamics of *tanha*, perhaps attempting to answer questions like, "What is this person pursuing?" or "What is this person attempting to avoid?" And we in doing so, we see the Second Noble Truth manifesting itself quite clearly in our patients and in ourselves.

One example of this appeared in the case of Rodney, a 36-year-old man who struggled with anger for several years following a painful divorce that involved losing primary custody of his children, who were being cared for by his wife and her new husband. Using a CFT "multiple selves" intervention in which the client explores the perspectives of different emotions and the patterns of attention, feelings, thoughts, motivations, and behaviors that accompany them, Rodney was *very able* to dive into exploration of his "angry self": "My anger feels strong and powerful. It helps me keep things together, and keep people away. To hell with them—they don't understand me!" Unfortunately, the way Rodney's chronic irritability and anger had manifested themselves in his life had distanced him further from his children, friends, and coworkers, and had created real problems in his job, which required him to be able to interact actively with other people. When it came time to explore other emotions, like anxiety and sadness, things turned out very differently: "I don't go there! I don't feel that stuff at all. I don't let myself—I push it away." Initially resistant to even explore these emotions, when finally asked, "What if you did let yourself feel anxiety? What would that be like? What thoughts would your anxious self think?" Rodney was able to connect: "I'd be terrified and feel weak. What if my kids love this other guy more than me? What if I lose my connection with them completely? I can't even allow myself to think about that stuff. I'm scared I'd completely fall apart." Shrinking in his chair, Rodney found his sadness even more difficult to explore: "That's where I never let myself go. If my sadness could talk, it would say that my life is ruined, and that it's my fault—that I destroyed the lives of everyone in the world that I love. I'd just want to lay down and die." Rodney then spontaneously put the pieces together: "That's what my anger is about! Every time I start to feel that stuff, I make myself mad—tell myself that this all happened because my wife is such a bitch, or think about how much I hate that jerk she's married. I like the anger. It feels powerful, like I'm in control. That other stuff—I can't take that other stuff. I'm scared that if I let myself go there, I might never get back."

Many of the ways we pursue our desires or attempt to avoid discomfort create great suffering for us. It is not as though craving appetitive stimuli and wishing to avoid aversives are "bad" in themselves. In Buddhist psychology, just as in behavior therapy, we are looking at the function of a behavior in context.

The truth of *tanha* suggests that our suffering is often driven by the domination of craving and avoidance-based behaviors. Just as a behavior therapist might, the Buddha examined these behaviors and their functions, and framed an intervention.

In accord with the historical Buddha's realization, the current state of the art of cognitive and behavioral research has established that excessive attempts at cognitive suppression or avoidance of unwanted mental events most often serves to increase the frequency of such events, and may intensify the distress with which they are experienced (Hayes, Follette, & Linehan, 2004; Wenzlaff & Wegner, 2000). The literature on the suppression of *expressing* our emotions may indicate that an adaptively flexible pattern of emotional responding may be useful—for example, choosing whether or not to express one's emotions given how helpful that may be in a particular context (Bonanno et al., 2004; Wilson & DuFrene, 2008). However, it has become clear that experiential avoidance can become a pervasive and ineffective regulation strategy and may play a role in the development, maintenance, or exacerbation of psychopathology (Campbell-Sills, Barlow, Brown, & Hofmann, 2006; Chapman, Gratz, & Brown, 2006; Hayes, Strosahl, & Wilson, 2011; Hayes et al., 2004; Kashdan, Breen, & Julian, 2010).

Experiential avoidance results when an individual is unwilling to accept or remain with a particular experience and takes steps to alter its form, frequency, or context (Hayes et al., 1996). Thus, experiential avoidance becomes a negatively reinforced strategy or response tendency that aims to reduce or end a distressing internal experience by avoiding or suppressing these private events, and is maintained through the process of escape conditioning (Chapman et al., 2006). These response tendencies can take many different forms aimed at escape or modification of a particular environmental or private event (Chapman et al., 2006). Individuals who frequently utilize experiential avoidance often engage in evasion, suppression, or other control tactics to manage or eliminate unwanted or distressful experiences such as thoughts, feelings, and somatic sensations (Campbell-Sills et al., 2006). Additionally, there is evidence to suggest that these individuals also engage in more verbal strategies to regulate their emotions (Cochrane, Barnes-Holmes, Barnes-Holmes, Stewart, & Luciano, 2007).

Such avoidance may provide short-term relief, but can lead to long-term detriment in functioning (Hayes et al., 1996). The negative effects of experiential avoidance result from the often ineffective and paradoxical self-perpetuating cycle of avoidance behaviors themselves (Hayes et al., 2004). For example, thought suppression and emotional avoidance can increase or prevent the extinction of an unwanted experience, disrupt emotional processing, and inadvertently strengthen the emotional response and/or the avoidant behavior (Abramowitz, Tolin, & Street, 2001; Campbell-Sills et al., 2006; Wenzlaff & Wegner, 2000). Habitual use of suppression or avoidance in response to emotional experiences has been associated with heightened levels of negative affect, lower levels of positive affect, poorer recovery from negative affect, poorer social adjustment, and decreased well-being (Campbell-Sills et al., 2006; Gross & John, 2003). Experiential avoidance has been hypothesized to function as a causal factor in a variety of psychological disorders: substance abuse (Forsyth, Parker, & Finlay, 2003), generalized anxiety disorder (Roemer, Orsillo, & Salters-Pedneault, 2008), panic disorder (White, Brown, Somers, & Barlow, 2006), postraumatic stress disorder (Kashdan et al., 2010; Marx & Sloan, 2005), and deliberate self-harm behavior (Chapman et al., 2006).

There are clear points of common ground between Buddhist psychology and behavioral research on the negative effects of experiential avoidance. However, the resonance between CBT and Buddhist psychology can also be viewed in terms of the work of the information-processing, or cognitivist, wing of the CBT community. Pioneering cognitive therapists, such as Aaron T. Beck (1976), based their theories on an observation that is similar to the insight expressed in the Buddha's Second Noble Truth: that it is not merely the things that happen to us that cause our suffering or mental illness, but what we make of them in our minds that makes the difference (Epstein, 1995). For example, Albert Ellis (2006) highlighted how the tendency to attach and cling to ideas about how we think things should be often manifests in the form of irrational thoughts that set us up for distress and disappointment. He observed that much of our distress results from thinking that things "must" be a certain way, or that we "should" do certain things, which leads us to discount positive situations and successes, and causes problems for us when things aren't the way we think they "must" be, or when we or others don't do the things we "should." The classic Ellis quotes regarding "musturbatory thinking" or "shoulding on yourself," as well as the Beckian emphasis on responding to irrational conditional assumptions, reflect a clear-eyed apprehension of the truth of *tanha*.

This emphasis is also rather directly reflected in the theory of cognitive dissonance (Festinger, 1957), describing the tendency for human beings to experience distress when we are confronted with observations about ourselves and the world that are inconsistent with our beliefs, such as when we observe ourselves behaving in ways that conflict with our values.

For thousands of years, the insight of the Second Noble Truth has influenced the development of Buddhist methods to address and alleviate human suffering. Over the last 20 years or so, third-wave behavior therapies, such as ACT, have developed empirically validated methods to address the components of experiential avoidance and psychological inflexibility, while identifying the core, measurable psychological processes that are involved in freedom from *dukkha* and *tanha*. As we set out together, we will explore this liberatory science as an extension of the *dharma*, and an advancement of the human experiment.

The Second Noble Truth establishes that the experience of suffering is an effect, one that is produced by causes. The Third Noble Truth makes the logical leap that if the causes can be identified, and if they can be affected, we can change the effect. The Third Noble Truth is the truth of liberation from suffering.

The Third Noble Truth: Liberation from Suffering

The Third Noble Truth states that we can free ourselves from *dukkha*, that human beings can liberate themselves from suffering. Most of us have heard the term *nirvana* which "etymologically means extinction of thirst and annihilation of suffering" (Das, 1997, p. 85). The Third Noble Truth tells us that it is possible to find peace, to weaken and ultimately overcome the cravings and attachment that cause so much of our suffering. The state of nirvana is often characterized by what it does not contain: obsession with our desires, powerful cravings that compel us in irrational ways, a reflexive and compulsive drive to avoid or escape experiences that we may view as unpleasant (Rahula, 1959/1974). The Third Noble Truth tells us that peace is possible. It's important to acknowledge that this state of liberation from craving is not one of passive neutrality; it isn't a lack of preferences or failing to address injustice, for example (Das, 1997). Rather, the liberation from craving described in the Third Noble Truth is seen as freeing us from the suffering and distractions caused by craving and clinging, so that we can act skillfully—much as the novice therapist must learn to free him- or herself from constant self-monitoring and self-evaluation in the therapy room before he or she can effectively implement treatment with his or her patients.

The Buddha felt that this message of hope—that finding peace was possible—was so important that he included it as one of his Noble Truths. There is a lesson in this that reverberates across successful forms of psychotherapy. Patients having positive expectations of therapy outcome has long been recognized as an important variable in psychotherapy, although it is often relegated to the status of a "nonspecific treatment effect" that must be controlled for in establishing the efficacy of new treatments (Kazdin, 1979). More recently, attention has been specifically paid to the role of hope as a positive motivation for change based on the combination of agency (the belief that one can begin and sustain movement toward a goal) and pathways (the belief that there are workable routes to the attainment of these goals) (Snyder et al., 2000). Research has provided evidence that this twofold operationalization of hope can predict better psychotherapy outcomes across stages of therapy (Irving et al., 2004). Like the Buddha, we need to find ways to give our patients both a pathway to improvement that they can believe in, and the sense that, with our help, this is something they can do.

While those of us who practice CBT may tend to avoid terms like "nirvana" and "enlightenment" in describing our treatment goals, we clearly attempt to free our patients from the tyranny of obsessive thoughts and of habitual behavioral tendencies that trap our patients in cycles of depression and anxiety (Dowd & McCleary, 2007; Dunn, Hartigan, & Mikulas, 1999; Hayes, Orsillo, & Roemer, 2010).

Contextual CBT, such as ACT, is based upon a psychological flexibility model (Hayes et al., 2006). This model emphasizes the whole person cultivating several central capacities that can increase clients' adaptive flexibility and their ability to respond to events in the present moment, in effective ways. Psychological flexibility represents a capacity to contact the present moment, with all that it contains, with a willingness to experience the full range of human emotions and experiences. It includes a capacity to hold our stories lightly, and to view the world and ourselves from a flexible and compassionate perspective, as we define and clarify patterns of action that grant our lives purpose, meaning, and vitality, committing to return to such valued directions in the face of the range of challenges that life presents (Hayes et al., 2011). While this aim does not have some of the assumptions that accompany some forms of Buddhism, this sense of liberation, of waking up to reality just as it is, and living in accordance with deeply held, perhaps universal, values is completely harmonious with the aims of Buddhist psychology.

Many of the techniques found in ACT and the cognitive-behavioral therapies are consistent with the Buddha's prescription for the alleviation of suffering, with examples including the activation of adaptive behavioral responses, assisting patients in decoupling from maladaptive patterns of thinking and learning more adaptive alternatives, or helping patients change their relationship to such thoughts so that they no longer accept them as true. The treatment goals of more recent cognitive-behavioral models seem to map even more closely onto the Buddhist pursuit of freedom from suffering.

For example, CFT (Gilbert, 2010a) considers the powerful tendencies of attachment and aversion as reflecting the activity of evolved emotion regulation systems, and utilizes specific behavioral, affective, cognitive, and imagery-based strategies to assist patients in developing the capacity to shift out of such modes of processing by (for example) activating emotion-regulation systems that produce a felt sense of peace and calm, help to balance our affective responding, broaden our attentional capacity, and enhance our cognitive flexibility (Gilbert, 2010c). Like the Buddha, we realize that freedom from suffering is not attainable simply by surrounding ourselves with luxuries, making the world around us perfect, or avoiding the inevitable pain and discomfort of life. To do so would be impossible, and wouldn't address the fundamental causes of suffering even were we to succeed. Rather, we can work to free ourselves by working with the degrees of freedom we have available to us—our capacities for behavior, thought, reasoning, and interaction—which brings us to the Buddha's Fourth Noble Truth, which is known as the path to the cessation of suffering (Succito, 2010) or the "Middle Path."

Clinical Example

Let's return to the client we met earlier, Rita, to take a look at how these first three truths can help us alleviate and prevent the suffering we encounter in others and in ourselves. To remind ourselves of these first three truths, they state:

- that life involves suffering;
- that suffering emerges from our craving to have what we cannot have, and to rid ourselves of what is unavoidable; and
- that we can train our minds to get out from under the dominance of craving and desire to escape, and this state of mind can free us from suffering.

We will look at one of Rita's earliest sessions, as her therapist used Buddhist-informed CBT to help create a context for change. Practitioners of a variety of cognitive and behavioral therapies might recognize elements of their way of working. For example, cognitive therapists will notice the Socratic questioning involved, and how the therapist and client look at the utility of her automatic thoughts together. ACT practitioners might notice that the therapist and client are engaging in a practice known as "creative hopelessness." In a creative hopelessness practice, the therapist gradually helps the client to notice the unworkability of attempts to excessively control or avoid unwanted inner experiences. CFT practitioners will likely notice the practice of "empathic bridging" and the "wisdom of no blame," as the therapist actively takes the affective perspective of the client, experiences the world through his or her eyes as much as he or she can, and reflects that the suffering the client has endured has not been freely chosen. Also, the practice of visualizing a compassionate version of the self will be demonstrated. DBT practitioners may notice the dyad sitting inside a dialectic of accepting difficult feelings and finding motivation for change. All CBT practitioners will likely notice the guided discovery and collaborative agenda setting that is at play. Importantly, such a session takes place in a context of mindful compassion, with the therapist slowing down, engaging the client with flexible, focused attention and a commitment to help them alleviate and prevent their suffering.

Rita has experienced panic attacks, flashbacks, nightmares, and persistent intrusive thoughts about the series of medical traumas that she endured throughout years of treatment for chronic illness as a child. Both of her parents struggled with anxiety disorders and addictions throughout her life, and she has very few memories of being adequately soothed or attended to, by either of her parents. She has met with the therapist to discuss her history and understands the foundations of a contextual and compassionate CBT model of treatment of PTSD. As they are beginning their work, Rita voices her concerns to her therapist. If this intervention sounds like the therapy you are doing, that is probably because it is in some ways, and because we are refining our methods together as a modern CBT community to access the wisdom we come into the world with, just like this client.

CLIENT: So, I do want to talk about something that is kind of embarrassing today.

THERAPIST: What might that be?

CLIENT: I get that all of this is "evidence-based" therapy and all that. I mean, that is why I'm here to see you. But I just don't believe that I'm going to get any better. I don't think this is going to work.

THERAPIST: Well, there is a lot of wisdom in that, you know?

CLIENT: What?

THERAPIST: I think that the part of you that says "This won't work." Maybe it has some wisdom.

CLIENT: Are you supposed to say that?

THERAPIST: Good question. I think it is okay for me to say that. What do you think?

CLIENT: It's okay with me. *(Pauses.)* In fact it is kind of a relief, but what do you mean "wisdom"? I just don't believe anything is going to work.

THERAPIST: Very good. Of course you don't. What does that feel like for you?

CLIENT: I don't know.

THERAPIST: Could you give the feeling a name?

CLIENT: I'm not sure. No.

THERAPIST: Where in your body do you feel something associated with this feeling?

CLIENT: I guess in my throat. I feel sort of "choked up," you know? And in my eyes, like I could cry.

THERAPIST: And what do you call that feeling?

CLIENT: Saaad. I'm really sad about this. Because I really want something to work, and there are so many scary memories and I just want them to go away.

THERAPIST: I don't blame you. I wish they would go away too, you know. If that was my job, it would be awesome. You come to me with these painful feelings, and I get to just make them all go away. That would feel pretty cool. Wish that worked, sort of.

CLIENT: *(Laughs.)* But, yeah . . . it doesn't just go away.

THERAPIST: What have you tried so far, you know, to make these feelings and memories go away?

CLIENT: I was in analysis for years, and that was interesting, but things only got worse. And then I used to just go out to bars and drink a lot, and that didn't help either.

THERAPIST: Not at all?

CLIENT: Well, it was fun and I had friends *(laughs)* but I couldn't stop the flashbacks and fear that way.

THERAPIST: What else have you tried?

CLIENT: I used to compulsively exercise, and I joined a human potential kind of group, you know, sort of a cult, but not really. . . .

THERAPIST: I think I know the kind of thing you mean . . .

CLIENT: But none of that helped. For a bit, maybe, but none of it really helped.

THERAPIST: Has anything really worked so far?

CLIENT: NO! That is what I'm saying. *(suddenly somewhat angry)* I just can't stop feeling this stuff. The flashbacks and the nightmares all suck. I can't stop being reminded of the pain no matter how much I try. I can't stop myself having panic attacks at all. Prozac didn't really stop them. I don't want to take benzos. Nothing can stop these feelings, and now I can't even get out of my dumb little apartment. I miss having friends. So, I can't believe that you are going to be able to help me. I'm sorry but I can't believe it.

THERAPIST: *There* is the wisdom that I was talking about. Maybe your mind is telling you something important here. Maybe you have just had so much that has caused you pain and fear, and you have tried so hard to rid yourself of it, and nothing has worked. So, every single effort you have had to avoid, kick away, or knock out these emotions has failed. The more you try to escape, control, and struggle, the more you are back where you began. I think your mind is correct here in a way, maybe we can't stop your feelings. It isn't your fault that you have wound up here, and maybe we just can't obliterate what you have felt, no matter what.

CLIENT: Okay, so this is weird, but I'm not freaked out by that idea.

THERAPIST: How do you mean?

CLIENT: You are telling me that we might not be able to stop me feeling panicky, and I would think that would freak me out, but it kind of doesn't right now. Is that weird?

THERAPIST: Not to me. No. It makes perfect sense, really. I think that, maybe, you have been fighting the wrong fight these years. Let's look at the thought that you have had about how to successfully deal with these problems. If you had to sum up your approach to your anxiety and trauma memories, what would it be?

CLIENT: Okay, this is one of those "automatic thoughts" or "beliefs" I read about in that cognitive therapy book, so the thought I have about my PTSD is that "I need to get rid of my PTSD symptoms, or it is going to ruin my life."

THERAPIST: Wow. You are a quick study. You came to work today, Rita! Very cool. So, if we think of the costs versus the benefits of you believing that, the costs versus the benefits of you buying into the idea "I need to get rid of my PTSD symptoms, or it is going to ruin my life!" What would we say the benefits are?

CLIENT: Hmmm . . . I am sorry to say that I can't think of any. Maybe that it keeps me motivated to get better? Maybe that, but nothing else really.

THERAPIST: So, believing that you have to reduce the symptoms of this "disorder" you have has fueled your motivation, but nothing else? Nothing at all?

CLIENT: It is like I said, I have gone from treatment to treatment, from prescription drugs to drinking too much, to eventually hiding from everybody. Nothing has worked.

THERAPIST: So we can see some more of this wisdom, can't we? What has it cost you, believing that you need to get rid of PTSD before you can have your life begin? What has it cost you to believe this thought?

CLIENT: Well, I've hidden from my friends and family. I can't go anywhere in case I have a panic attack. I don't work now. It has cost me just about everything that I love in life. I'm all alone.

THERAPIST: Honestly, Rita, I'm very sad to hear that. I get it. I really want to thank you for bringing me that much closer to what this is like for you. Your life has gotten so much smaller. It would mean something to me to help you get your life back.

CLIENT: Yes. I want my life back.

THERAPIST: I want you to have that too. I really do. If we could do something really different to help you reclaim your life. Would you be willing to try?

CLIENT: I'm not sure.

THERAPIST: Well, that is some awesome honesty. Let's do a little perspective exercise with this, okay?

CLIENT: Why not.

THERAPIST: Thanks. Let's imagine that it is 60 years from now, and you have gone on struggling to make your PTSD go away. You have had a few victories, but just like you said, mostly nothing worked. You have, however, continued to grow into a very loving person. You were very loving to your mom and dad, even though they failed you. You were an amazing aunt to the nephew you love so much. You were always there for the friends that you kept. People thought of you as a really caring and giving person. But you were so afraid to step out into the world, so afraid of triggers, that you mostly just hid from the world. So, you are 95 now, and it is getting to feel like it is near the end. An old friend visits you, and she tells you she has an amazing app for her smartphone, or watch, or supercomputer chip in your head (you know it is far in the future). They have a time machine. So, this buddy of yours spins a wheel and this compassionate, wise, and caring future self goes back in time. And right here in that spare chair, right now, with us, this loving future version of yourself is sitting there. She looks you in your eyes and she sees all of the pain there, and she knows how things turn out for you if you continue to avoid facing your fears and living your life.

I want you to sit in this open chair. *(Client moves to the chair.)* Look into the chair where the Rita today is sitting. *(pause)* Before you do, I want you to breathe in and out slowly, with care. *(pause)* Release excess tension with each breath. *(pause)* Now open your eyes, and with a voice of wisdom, strength, and commitment, tell Rita what she needs to know to live her life fully. You can do it. . . .Tell her.

CLIENT: *(After a pause, and after a few deep breaths she looks at the empty chair.)* Rita, you poor, poor girl. I'm so sorry for what you have been through. Still, this is the only life you have, dear. This is it. When it is gone, we are done. Please, please don't let it slip away. If you need to have help, get that help, but don't keep fighting this way. You can live your life. It is worth it. You can live your life.

THERAPIST: Very good. Do you see all that wisdom that was wrapped inside your pain? Wow!

CLIENT: I don't know where that came from. *(Moves back to her chair.)*

THERAPIST: Do you think in the next weeks we can, maybe, begin to find a way to step forward in your life, even with the pain? Do you think we could aim for that together?

CLIENT: Yes. I believe we can. I don't know what will happen, but it . . . it feels okay, it feels safe enough . . . to just aim for that . . . to have my life back. You know? Is this crazy? I think we can.

THERAPIST: You didn't ask for any of this, and it is actually an honor to step forward with you. It is going to mean a lot of change and it might be really tough. Are you willing to aim for this together?

CLIENT: Yes, actually. Yes I am.

The Fourth Noble Truth: The Middle Path Intervention

While the first three foundational principles of Buddhist psychology represent processes at work in the self and in the world, the Fourth Noble Truth provides us with an intervention strategy. The Middle Path goes farther than the prior prescriptions of the historical Buddha in that it makes direct suggestions for specific steps in the alleviation of suffering. This path is often referred to as the "Noble Eightfold Path," as it involves eight capacities that the student of Buddhism will strive to develop. We will outline this path, and in doing so, it will become clear to you that the historical Buddha was actually clearly delineating a methodical, replicable, cognitive and behavioral intervention, one that had the explicit aim of helping people to alleviate their suffering. As this is a book that aims to place the Buddhist perspective squarely into a secular and clinical CBT context, we are going to refer to the Fourth Noble Truth as the "Middle Path intervention." As we encounter each dimension of the Eightfold Path, we will provide examples of contemplative, clinical applications that relate to this aspect of the Fourth Noble Truth. These techniques will be drawn from both Buddhist psychology and CBT. We would also like to invite you to consider how you might improvise, invent, and adapt new techniques to train the mind in the various capacities of the Middle Path intervention.

The Middle Path
and Adaptive Conduct

> You can hold yourself back from the sufferings of
> the world, that is something you are free to do and
> it accords with your nature, but perhaps this very
> holding back is the one suffering you could avoid.
> —FRANZ KAFKA

Although the scientific method, as such, had not been developed when Siddartha Gotama lived, we have in Buddhist psychology a powerful forerunner of applied psychological science that may contain not only the roots, but also the branches that will develop into our cognitive-behavioral theories, technologies, and traditions. The Fourth Noble Truth—the Eightfold Path—is a step-by-step series of practices that can be empirically explored by any individual, acting as their own scientist practitioner. Accordingly, the Eightfold Path of Buddhist practice is more of a road map of adaptive and flexible response patterns to life's challenges than it is a series of commandments, laws, or strictures based on religious assumptions. Here we present them in the guise of the Middle Path intervention.

THE MIDDLE PATH INTERVENTION

The method that is delineated in the Middle Path intervention guides the Buddhist practitioner in developing specific capacities that are designed to produce a happy, peaceful life, which may propel one on toward eventual liberation from suffering. While many of the components of the Eightfold Path offer specific prohibitions concerning speech, behavior, and actions, these prohibitions are based on the assertion that certain ways of acting tend to cause harm and difficulty, and interfere with functioning. The question is not so much "ethical" in the conventional sense of the word, but of what is workable if one's aim is the alleviation of suffering. Accordingly, we will be using the term "adaptive" rather than the term "ethical," and the term "healthy" rather than the term "right" throughout our presentation of the Middle Path intervention for CBT clinicians. While Buddhist scholars and language experts might find these substitutions to be out of step with earlier translations, our approach aims to be a workable adaptation of a flexible, living tradition for the purposes we are looking to serve.

The eight steps of the Buddhist psychology approach are often presented in three general categories (Rahula, 1959/1974). This classification system can make the sequence and implementation of these elements clearer to us as we set upon the Eightfold Path. We can consider the three categories—adaptive conduct, mental discipline, and wisdom—to be three aspects of liberation from suffering. This chapter and the next will introduce these three categories, and provide experiential practices to contact and embody the elements of the Eightfold Path. These practices are by no means the only way to realize the elements of the Middle Path intervention, and they are not all part of the orthodox body of formal Buddhist practice. Each of the eight elements of the Middle Path can be realized through virtually limitless combinations of human behavior, with all such variations converging on one point of intention: the alleviation of human suffering. This chapter introduces the elements of adaptive conduct: healthy speech, healthy action, and healthy livelihood.

HEALTHY SPEECH

"Healthy speech" in Buddhist psychology involves speaking truthfully, kindly, meaningfully, and helpfully, and generally refraining from forms of speech that do not meet these criteria. With healthy speech, we use our verbal behavior to communicate clearly and genuinely: we don't tell lies, or attempt to confuse or mislead. Whether we are directing audible words to others, or having a mental discussion with ourselves, healthy speech involves speaking from a compassionate perspective, and refraining from cruelty, gossip, or comments designed to directly or indirectly intimidate, promote distress, discomfort, or hard feelings. Healthy speech is helpful, designed to facilitate positive outcomes, in the way that good psychotherapy is—it can be helpfully critical but not judgmental, involving what Paul Gilbert (2010a) refers to as compassionate correction rather than shameful attacking. Healthy speech also involves eschewing what Buddhists term "idle speech," banter or gossip that serves little purpose but to distract the mind from more meaningful, adaptive pursuits.

Traditionally, healthy speech has stood for the conduct of our overt verbal behavior, meaning the actual words we use when speaking aloud to others. We can imagine a range of CBT techniques and directions that are useful in developing healthy speech; these include the interpersonal effectiveness skills found in DBT (Linehan, 1993a, 1993b), John Gottman's principles for effective communication in couple therapy (1999), and training in assertive communication. All of these techniques may be useful in developing healthy speech, from a Buddhist psychology perspective. However, the concept of speech may also extend to the type of cognition that is often targeted in CBT: "self-talk." As we extend and adapt the principles of the Eightfold Path to cognitive behavioral practice, we can explore how moving toward healthy self-directed speech can be enacted as an aim for treatment.

Cognitive-behavioral researchers have repeatedly found that self-critical and debasing self-talk is related to negative psychological outcomes (Dunkley, Zuroff, & Blankstein, 2003, 2006; Rector, Bagby, Segal, Joffe, & Levitt, 2000; Sachs-Ericsson, Verona, Joiner, & Preacher, 2006). Indeed, much of the focus of Beckian cognitive therapy involves identifying potentially psychologically harmful self-talk and deliberately reframing our internal verbal responses in more rational, balanced, or helpful words (Dobson, 2009; Hofmann, 2012). Just as cognitive therapy focuses often on cognitive content, ACT often involves patients and therapists working together to understand the function of emotionally distressing, internal verbal behaviors. ACT employs experiential and relational techniques that can help a patient to realize how his or her cognitions and negative self-talk exerts a powerful, dominant influence upon his or her state of mind and range of available behaviors. Rather than addressing the content for specific change, ACT encourages patients to loosen the grip that such mental events may have upon them, by seeing thoughts for what they are, rather than responding to thoughts as though they were literal events. As the Buddhist Nun Thubten Chodron has asserted in a recent book title, both Buddhist psychology and CBT suggest, "Don't believe everything you think" (2012). As such, healthy speech involves our understanding that the words we use with ourselves, as well as with others, carry strong influences upon our behavior and emotions. By bringing mindfulness, acceptance, and compassion to our speech, we are following the Eightfold Path, and moving towards liberation of suffering in both Buddhist psychology and CBT terms.

Compassionate Letter Writing

Part of healthy speech involves connecting with the aspects of yourself that directly contribute to your well-being. Different emotional states and experiences will, of course, influence our thoughts and our words. For example, if you imagine that you are at a job interview with a seemingly hostile and impatient employer, at a time when you really need the job, what self-talk might you experience, and what words might you say? Alternatively, if you imagine that you are holding your firstborn child close to you, and looking into his or her eyes with love, what might you think and say? Compassion-focused approaches to CBT, such as CFT (Gilbert, 2010c) seek to stimulate emotional systems that generate positive affiliative emotions that can lead to adaptive self-talk and conduct. Just as a method actor can use imagination to "get into character" and speak from another perspective, the following CFT exercise will involve training yourself to access the most supportive parts of you, and to speak from this place. This exercise will include you writing a letter to yourself with a deeply compassionate, wise, and unconditionally accepting voice. This voice is intended to express the innate loving-kindness, strength, and intuitive wisdom that we all have as part of our basic humanity.

Practices that seek to help cultivate self-compassion are particularly useful with clients with shame-based difficulties and self-criticism. How many of us practicing CBT have found that our clients could understand how to "rationally" challenge their inner critics, but could not access emotional states of warmth and self-kindness. Letter writing and imagery exercises offer our clients a way to deliberately stimulate their experience of self-forgiveness and compassion, creating a context for emotional and behavior change.

Guided Instructions

To prepare, set aside some time when you can engage in this exercise mindfully. Find a space that feels comfortable and safe, and bring a paper, pen, and surface to write on.

As you begin, allow your eyes to close. Now, gently direct your attention to the sounds around you in the room. When you are ready, after several seconds, bring your attention to the sounds outside of the room. Next, direct your attention to the sounds even farther away than that. On the next inhalation, allow your attention to gently gather at the level of physical sensation. When you are ready, bring your awareness to the movement of the breath in the abdomen. Observe whatever sensations are present in the abdomen, allowing your attention to collect and gather on the inhalation, and letting go of the awareness of particular sensations as you exhale. Allow this breath to flow in its own rhythm. Beyond this, allow yourself to settle into this awareness, abiding in a state of bare observation, suspending judgment, evaluation, or even description. It is the nature of our minds to wander and drift away from the breath. When we notice this drift of attention, we may even briefly acknowledge ourselves for having a moment of self-awareness, and gently return our attention to the flow of the breath.

After spending some time with mindful breathing, allow your attention to rest on the flow of your thoughts as you inhale. Letting go of the attention to the breath, bring your current life situation to mind. What conflicts, problems, or self-criticisms come to mind? Where is your attention pulled? What is your mind beginning to tell you? What changes occur in your body? What emotions arise within you? What images reveal themselves in your mind?

As you exhale, intentionally let go. On the next available in-breath direct your attention to an image of yourself as a compassionate and wise being. Imagine yourself as kind, as emotionally strong and resilient, and as a loving and accepting presence. In your compassionate mind, you possess wisdom and emotional strength. You are unconditionally accepting of all that you are, in this moment, and are completely noncondemning. Your compassionate self radiates emotional warmth and wisdom. This is the voice that you will be bringing to your letter writing today. You will be writing from the perspective of this understanding, self-accepting, broad perspective. In this way, we are contacting a wisdom that you were born with, and giving it a voice. For a moment, recognize the calmness and wisdom that you possess. Take a moment to feel the physical sensations that company the arising of a compassionate mind. Recognize the strength and healing quality of a vast and deep kindness. Recognize that this loving kindness, this powerful compassion exists within you as an abundant reservoir of strength. Take a moment to step back and observe the flow of thoughts and feelings that emerge moment by moment. Hold this process of unfolding mental events before you.

As you encounter this compassionate self, remember the simple act of self-validation. There are many good reasons for the distress you are currently experiencing. Your brain and mind have evolved and emerged through millions of years of life progressing on this planet. You were not designed to deal with the particular pressures and complexities of our current social environment. Your learning history has presented you with strong challenges, and situations that have caused you pain. Can you open yourself to a compassionate understanding that your struggle is a natural part of life, and that it is not your fault?

As much as you can, connect with the basic kindness and care that you would bring to a beloved friend. If you were writing this letter to a truly beloved friend, a person whom you held in great kindness, what would you want to say? What would you write in your letter? Wouldn't you validate your friend's suffering? Wouldn't you reach out to let him or her know that whatever he or she has done, he or she is are still worthy of love and kindness? Wouldn't you try to help him or her to find ways to take action, to move his or her life to a greater state of well-being and meaningfulness?

On the next exhale, slowly open your eyes and prepare to write. In the next few minutes, allow yourself to compose a compassionate letter that gives a voice to the most compassionate part of you. As you write, think about what compassionate actions you could take to help better your current situation. What kind of compassionate attention might you bring to your life right now? How can you be as understanding and patient as you can be with yourself? If you are working with a therapist, when you next meet with your therapist, if you feel willing, bring this letter to session. Together, you and your therapist can read and reflect upon the words and feelings that you have allowed yourself to express below. If you are working independently, set aside some time to mindfully read this letter back to yourself with great care. Let yourself hear the words and feel the emotional tone of compassion that you have written. If you feel the need to write drafts of this letter several times, please feel free to do this.

Based on compassionate letter-writing exercises developed by Gilbert (2009a), Tirch (2102), and Neff (2011).

HEALTHY ACTION

The concept of "healthy action" refers to adaptive overt behavior, in the most conventional understanding of the term "behavior." Fundamentally, healthy action involves behaving in ways that promote the well-being of self and others, ways that are basically kind and helpful. It also involves refraining from behaviors that cause harm. Healthy action involves refraining from a range of behaviors such as killing, doing harm, stealing, exploiting others, unbalancing the mind with intoxicants, or engaging in compulsive or psychologically damaging sexual practices (Rahula, 1959/1974). Healthy action also means acting in ways that are responsible and that promote the happiness of every being. For example, healthy action might involve practicing generosity and stewardship; having the courage to address social injustice; and working to protect those who are vulnerable, including ourselves (Nhat Hahn, 1998). According to Thich Nhat Hahn, healthy action is inextricably linked with mindfulness—paying attention in the present moment with acceptance (Germer, 2009). Human beings can all too easily become deluded about what the "right" thing to do is. Adherence to rule-governed behavior over and above a flexible values-based response to present moment consequences has been found to be correlated with a number of negative psychological outcomes in the contextual behavioral science literature (Hayes, Zettle, & Rosenfarb, 1989). Through effort justification and a fused perspective upon our behavioral attributions (Cerutti, 1989; Hayes, 2004a) human beings may find themselves convinced of the moral correctness of their actions. However, these actions may have much more to do with the influence of habitual patterns of avoidance and addictive craving than with behavior that is in the service of helping others and ourselves.

Taking the example of exposure in behavioral therapy, one can observe that from a naïve perspective, exposure therapy may look like a form of torture. A therapist is intentionally encouraging a person to remain in the direct presence of something that causes him or her great anxiety and distress. However, with awareness of how the human fear response works, we come to see exposure as a crucial component as we work to help our patients overcome debilitating anxiety (Barlow, 2004). Healthy action, in such a case, does not involve the pursuit of short-term gratification of appetitive cravings, or hiding from things that are frightening or aversive. Healthy action actually involves moving toward a source of anxiety, so that a person might eventually habituate to the experience, develop a greater fear tolerance, and cultivate a broader and more flexible range of adaptive behaviors in the presence of anxiety-provoking stimuli. Identification of healthy action involves mindfulness, flexibility in perspective taking, identification of what "healthy" means in a given context, and commitment to pursue this healthy action, even in the presence of difficult experiences. Contextual behavior science and contextual CBT suggest that all of these qualities can be deliberately developed. In this way CBT and Buddhist psychology appear to serve one another's shared aims, providing a range of methods to pursue adaptive behaviors and healthy actions, even when such behaviors may not immediately present themselves in obvious forms.

Enhancing Healthy Action through Pleasant Events

Healthy action involves taking those behavioral steps that will contribute to our well-being, even when destructive emotions or negatively biased thoughts tell us that we are better off remaining inactive. Anhedonia in depression, and a decrease in engagement in experiences of pleasure and mastery, can lead to insufficient rewards in a person's life and a restricted range of action (Beck, 1976). The pattern of depressed mood leading to isolation and inactivity and to deeper depression is likely all too familiar to the CBT clinician and depressed patient. Just as the Buddha's Eightfold Path would suggest, deeply engaging in healthy action can help liberate us from a downward spiral of depression and constricted lives.

Behavioral activation (BA) is a long-standing evidence-based CBT technique frequently used in the treatment of depression and other mood disorders (Martell, Addis, & Jacobson, 2001). In particular, BA has been found to be the essential component in CBT treatment of acute depression, demonstrating results that are superior to medication or cognitive interventions in some important randomized controlled trials (Jacobson et al., 1996; Jacobson, Martell, & Dimidjian, 2001).

In its most basic form, BA can involve a patient increasing his or her engagement in experiences of pleasure and mastery. In order to facilitate this change, CBT therapists often provide their patients with a form of schedule, that they can use to record their actions throughout the day each day, assessing each activity for how rewarding it may be. As patients become more aware of what activities involve pleasure and mastery, regardless of what the depressed mind may forecast, the hope is that they will increase their engagement, and engage in more rewarding experiences, reversing the spiral of depression.

It stands to reason that bringing mindful, flexible, and focused attention to present moment experience might help with the processes involved in BA. Accordingly, MBCT (Segal, Williams, & Teasdale, 2012) an empirically supported, mindfulness-based intervention for depressive relapse, has developed a particular form of BA that embodies the qualities of healthy action in the Middle Path.

A "Pleasant Events Calendar" (see Figure 3.1) is used in MBCT to guide patients in the practice of directing their attention to positive events and the emotional experiences connected to activities in their lives (Crane, 2009). The MBCT Pleasant Events Calendar can be used to bring applied mindfulness to everyday pleasant events, deepening the experience of the moment rather than simply evaluating the levels of pleasure and mastery on a numerical scale. The experiences recorded on the calendar include emotions, physical sensations, and thoughts both during and after a pleasant event. An example of a structured Pleasant Events Calendar is provided below.

This exercise can help patients cultivate full attention and awareness of their experience of healthy action. In clinical practice, a CBT practitioner may choose to introduce mindfulness exercises before using this Pleasant Events Calendar. However, a clinician might also introduce the quality of mindfulness by gently walking through the series of questions that are on the calendar in a session with the patient, preparing him or her to use this calendar as a homework practice. In such a way, the evidence-based processes involved in BA, in mindfulness, and in an empathically attuned psychotherapy relationship can all be activated. The following introduction is an example of this approach:

"I'd like to introduce you to a new way that we can practice bringing deliberate, accepting attention to the positive events and activities in your life. Now, we both know that during depression, our minds can be tricky, and can discourage us from believing that we will enjoy those things that have brought us pleasure and well-being in the past. Let's practice how deliberately paying attention can

This week, be aware of one pleasant event, activity, or occurrence each day *while it is happening.* As you bring mindful awareness to this event or activity, answer the questions that follow below. Increasing awareness and engagement can bring us closer to healthy action, and to the freedom to choose lives that involve a greater sense of purpose, meaning, and even pleasure in our daily lives.

Date	Event Details	Physical Sensations	Feelings or emotions	When did you become aware of these feelings? During? After?	Thoughts or images at the time of the event?	Thoughts now as you record this experience?

FIGURE 3.1. Pleasant Events Calendar

help us engage more deeply with healthy action. Think of one pleasant event, no matter how small, and we will work through the questions on this calendar together. Shall we begin?"

Adapted from material in Segal, Williams, and Teasdale (2012).

Clinical Example

For a clinical example involving healthy speech and action, let's return to the case of Rodney, whom we first met in Chapter 2. Having identified that his irritability and angry thoughts and behavior served to help him avoid more difficult, vulnerable feelings like anxiety and sadness, Rodney worked together with his therapist to develop other ways of approaching the antecedents to his problematic anger episodes. They identified the primary antecedents as including thoughts and feelings of estrangement from his children, self-criticism and shame over how his angry acting-out had created problems in his family and at work, and his considerable reluctance to feel anxiety and sadness. In the process of the CFT that Rodney and his therapist were working on, Rodney engaged in a good deal of compassionate-self work, which involves cultivating specific compassionate qualities, including helpful speech and action. These were explored in a later session of the therapy, in a perspective-taking exercise similar to the one we engaged in with our client Margaret.

THERAPIST: So when you look at this situation with your children from the kind, wise, confident perspective of your compassionate self, does it make sense that you would feel anger, anxiety, and sadness?

RODNEY: Of course it does! I can't imagine anything worse than losing your kids like this. I mean, I haven't lost them exactly, but it sure feels like it. It feels terrible.

THERAPIST: So you can understand where those angry, anxious, and sad selves are coming from?

RODNEY: Absolutely! I have so many feelings when I think about this stuff. It can be overwhelming.

THERAPIST: So here, from the perspective of this wise, kind, confident, compassionate self—who recognizes how difficult this situation is for you and others—what would you want to say to that part of you that is hurting so bad—feeling all of this anger, fear, and sadness? Imagine that you could have a private talk with that part of you that is hurting so terribly over this situation, and feeling all of these scary feelings. You are speaking to that part of you from a place of compassion and patience, just as we are speaking here together. Let yourself really see how bad that part of you is suffering, and really feel for him. What would you want to say to him? What would you want him to understand about how he's feeling? Like we did before, speak directly to him.

RODNEY: I would tell him that there's nothing wrong with him. Of course, you're going to feel all that stuff, and it doesn't make you crazy. You've made some mistakes, but you're really trying. This is really hard, what you're going through, but things will get better, and you can do things to help with that.

THERAPIST: What sort of things could he do, Rodney? What could he do that would help?

RODNEY: Well, he could call the kids more often. He wants to call them a lot, but then all those feelings come up and he doesn't. *(Becomes tearful, and turns to look at the therapist.)* I love them so much, and I need to let them know it. I need to stop letting this stuff get in my way and call them. I need to make sure that I follow through with the plans I've made with them, even though I hate going over to pick them up at their house. I need to make sure they know how I feel about them.

THERAPIST: It sounds like you want to connect with them and follow through, but something gets in the way. Could you tell me more about that?

RODNEY: I want to call them, but then I feel so terrible about not having been in touch as much as I should have that I stop. And I want to do things with them, but it feels so terrible going over there to pick them up—I see his mother and Derek [new husband], and that big house they have, and I'm alone in my apartment. I worry that the kids won't want to be around me, and that they're embarrassed of me.

THERAPIST: So you want to connect with them, but when you start to, all these thoughts and feelings come up that feel really threatening, so you back off.

RODNEY: They stop me in my tracks.

THERAPIST: So again from the perspective wisdom and compassion, how might you reassure yourself and encourage yourself to keep going?

RODNEY: Let me think. I guess I'd tell myself that the kids really do love you and enjoy spending time with you. Hell, even their mother will admit to that. So you can be a good Dad, no matter where you live. They need you, and you need them. You just need to reach out to them, even though it's hard. You've done it before. You have. And you can do it again. *(Turns straight to the therapist.)* God, I love them.

THERAPIST: Is there something you could do today that would be a step toward that?

RODNEY: I'm going to call them right after we're done and firm up plans for this weekend. This is my weekend and we haven't even made plans yet. We've been talking about going to see a ball-game. They both really like the games. I'm going to call and set that up with them.

THERAPIST: Sounds like a plan. Good work, Rodney. Good work.

HEALTHY LIVELIHOOD

Healthy livelihood involves extending the concept of healthy action to particularly emphasize how we materially support ourselves. By focusing on healthy livelihood, the historical Buddha is reminding us of the powerful effects that a vocation, career, craft, or trade can have upon our state of mind. Refraining from making a living in ways intentionally that cause harm to others is a foundational tenet of healthy livelihood. Of course, as the alleviation of suffering is an overt aim of Buddhist psychology, it would make sense that Buddhist practitioners would seek to support themselves in ways that did not cause harm. Historically, healthy livelihood has included avoiding careers that overtly cause harm to others, such as slave trading, arms dealing, or engaging in violence for money. This refraining has also been extended to trading in pornography and trading in alcohol or intoxicating drugs. Monastic Buddhists would also exclude careers that involve killing of any sort, such as hunting, fishing, or soldiering. However, there have been many lay Buddhist policemen and military service members over the centuries, as well as even warrior monks. Ultimately, those jobs that serve to exploit, sexualize, and delude us in pursuit of profit, or which desensitize us in ways that are harmful, could be viewed as opposed to healthy livelihood.

Importantly the Eightfold Path is designed as guidelines for positive personal practice, rather than as a metric for evaluating the actions of others. One can extend the concept of healthy livelihood to incorporate how one engages in any sort of career path one might pursue. The operative question in such cases involves the extent to which work practices allow for the alleviation of suffering, and do not contribute to uselessly causing harm. Being a psychotherapist may seem like an obvious road to healthy livelihood, but it is more than what one does, it is how one does it that constitutes healthy livelihood. So, in exploring our degree of healthy action we may ask ourselves hard questions. Below are some examples:

- As clinicians in private practice do we deal with others compassionately, or do we work to maximize business success over fully meeting the needs of our patients?
- Do we engage in business practices that have integrity?
- Do we pay more mind to providing our research assistants and postdoctoral fellows with experiences that will enhance their own training and viability as professionals?
- Are we grounding our psychotherapy in evidence-based principles and procedures, and staying current with developments in the research literature?
- How are we relating to the community of CBT and other professionals in our region?
- Are we maintaining self-care, and approaching our work in a way that is responsible to our patients, to our families, and to ourselves?

Asking these questions, and responding adaptively to what we find in the answers, requires attention, compassion, and wisdom, as it is easy to hold to our goals so firmly that we turn a blind eye to signs that our practices fail to reflect our values.

Sitting Inside Significant Questions

The contemporary protégé Tibetan meditation master, Yongey Mingyur Rinpoche has described mindfulness as "the key, the *how* of Buddhist practice [that] lies in learning to simply rest in bare awareness of thoughts, feelings and perceptions as they occur" (p. 43). This means that in addition to the practice of formal mindfulness meditation, we can activate our mindful awareness as we face the many challenges that life presents us. This application of mindfulness to the difficult questions of life can extend to how we approach the many problems that we face as 21st-century participants in our massively multitasking globalized society.

When we think of healthy livelihood as described in the Middle Path, we might limit the concept to just our careers, or how we make a living. However, each aspect of our lives in this era is essentially a part of our livelihood, just as a farmer in the Himalayas 2,600 years ago would basically be engaged in his vocation from dawn until dusk. ACT founder Kelly Wilson (Wilson & Dufrene, 2009) has designed a practice that consciously brings mindful awareness to the authorship of valued aims for our daily lives. Known as "sitting inside significant questions," this exercise involves evoking engaged mindfulness that is then deployed to address the big questions about how we wish to live our lives, and to what sort of a person we really wish to be. The exercise brings us face to face with our uncertainty and our ambivalence, as we gently wade out into the process of being the architect of a life of meaning, purpose, and vitality. We have adapted this practice below, as a part of our Middle Path intervention. It can take some time to work through, and, like the other practices in this book, you might want to refer to the audio exercise that guides you through the practice at *www.guilford. com/tirch-materials* as you engage with the meditation.

So many of our patients will come to us struggling as to how to find meaning in their lives and their work. The following practice can provide you with a bridge, developed from Buddhist psychology and CBT, that can help you walk with your patients toward healthy livelihood and well-being.

Finding the motivation to move in meaningful and purposeful directions is an important part of CBT for a range of psychological problems. Furthermore, increasing rewarding and self-affirming experiences is also an important part of CBT. We know of many examples of such techniques. As noted, seeking experiences of pleasure and mastery is a key part of CBT treatment of depression. Finding the motivation to engage in situational exposure is essential for the treatment of agoraphobia. Engaging in meaningful actions while tolerating distress plays a central role in CBT treatments for emotion regulation difficulties, such as DBT. ACT protocols for a range of problems such as anxiety, depression, trauma, and eating disorders all involve the authorship of valued aims. The following practice is compatible with all of these treatments and resonates with the Buddhist emphasis on mindful engagement in healthy livelihood.

Guided Instructions

In a few moments, if you are willing, I would like to offer you a guided exercise that focuses on those areas in your life that are most important to you. After we establish our practice, I will ask you a series of questions. You do not need to answer any of the questions; in fact, see if you can allow yourself just to linger in the questions, considering the experience of the question without acting upon the urge to answer or give in to dismay if you don't know the answer. Aim to simply reside in the question mark, in the uncertainty.

As you begin, allow your eyes to close. Now, gently direct your attention to the sensation of breathing. Noticing the way in which the breath feels in the body. Allowing the breath to flow in its own natural rhythm. Beyond this, allow yourself to settle into this awareness, abiding in a state of bare observation, suspending judgment, evaluation, or description.

I am going to ask you a sequence of questions about areas of your life. Some of these areas may seem significant and important to you while others may not. Listen to what is being asked, making room for each question. As best you can, adopt a curious and open awareness, noticing any thoughts, feelings, memories, or sensations that arise, and then return your awareness to pondering particular areas of your life. Simply sit with and appreciate these questions as questions. Allowing each question to be as it is, unanswered. When you find your mind coming up with answers or responses, gently release these thoughts and return to inhabiting the question.

Family: On the next inhale, I am going to ask you about the areas of family. What does being a family member mean to you? What kind of family member do you want to be? If something were to change in the area of family, what would that mean to you? Allow yourself to settle into these questions even if they do not feel significant for you, expanding your awareness around them and possibly out from them. On the next out-breath, let go of these question about family and return your attention to breathing.

Married couples, or intimate relations: Now I am going to focus questions on romantic relationships. What is important for you in romance and intimacy? What does being a romantic or intimate partner mean to you? What type of partner, wife, or lover do you want to be? What would it mean to you if something were to happen in these areas of your life? No matter how important these questions may feel, simply allow yourself to be with each of them. Sitting in and appreciating each question. On the next exhale, let go of these questions and gently return your attention to mindful breathing.

Parenting: With the next in-breath, ask yourself what does being a parent mean for you? What type of parent would you like to be? What if something were to change in the area of parenting? If you are not a parent, perhaps you can be with the inquiry as a way of imagining what the process of being a parent might be like for you. Continue to allow yourself to inhabit each question. On the next exhale, let go of these questions gently return your attention to breathing. Breathing in and breathing out.

Friends and social relations: Now with this breath, I am going to inquire about social life. What does friendship mean to you? What type of friend do you want to be? What changes would be meaningful to you in the areas of new friend and old friends? Allow yourself to settle into the entirety of each question, into their meaning. On the next exhale, let go of these questions and return your attention to the sensations of breathing.

Work: And now with the next in-breath, I will ask about what work means for you. What kind of employee or employer do you want to be? How do you want to work in a meaningful way? What would meaningful change in work be for you? Simply sit with these questions, expanding your awareness around them and possibly out from them. Sitting in the entirety of the meaning in each question. On the next exhale, let go of these questions and with the in-breath gently return your attention to breathing.

Education and training: With your next in-breath I will ask about meaningful learning. What does education and training mean to you? What approach to learning feels meaningful for you? What would expanding your knowledge or skills mean to you? Guide your awareness into and out from each of these questions, resting in their meaning and the question mark itself. Now, with the in-breath gently let go of these questions and bring your attention back to the breath.

Recreation, play, and fun: With the next in-breath, I invite you to ponder the area of recreation. What is meaningful fun and play? What is important recreation and relaxation? What if something meaningful were to happen in the area of play? Expand your awareness within and around each question and the unknown possibilities. On the next exhale, let go of these questions and return your focus to breathing.

Community life: With the next available in-breath, I will ask about community connections. What does community mean to you? What type of community member do you aim to be? What would it mean if something were to happen in the communities in your life? Again, gently expanding your awareness into and out from each of these questions, resting in their meaning and the nature of their inquiry. On the next exhale, let go of these questions and allow your attention to reside with the breath.

Spirituality: Now, gently bring your awareness to the area of spirituality. What does spirituality mean to you? What would it mean if something were to happen in the area of spirituality in your life? Even if these questions do not feel significant for you, or you have never considered them in this way before, simply allow yourself to sit with each question, as a question. On the next out-breath, let go of these questions and gently return your awareness to breathing.

Physical health and self-care: Now, I will ask about health and wellness. What does self-care mean for you? What would meaningful change be for you in the area of health? What is meaningful participation in wellness? Expand your awareness into and out from each of them, resting in their possible meaning and uncertainty. On the next exhale, let go of these questions and with the inhale allow your attention to reside with the breath.

On the next breath, begin to expand your awareness to include all these questions about the areas of your life: family, friendships, parenting, marriage and romance, spirituality, community, work, learning, health, play, and aesthetics.

After you have spent some time with this, gently allow your breath and attention to return to settle on the physical sensations in the abdomen. Now, with the next in-breath, allow your attention to focus on the sounds that surround you in the room. Next, bring the attention to the sounds outside of the room. Following this, allow your attention to gently settle on the sounds even farther away than that. Giving yourself a few moments to gather your attention and orientation to your presence on the mat, and when you feel ready, you can open your eyes.

Based on an exercise in Wilson and Dufrene (2009).

After completing this practice it can be helpful to make note of what you noticed. Keeping these areas of your life in mind, begin to write about what arises for you. What are the most important things in the areas and questions you sat with? Take 10 minutes or so to write down these meaningful things and why you feel they are important to you. See if you can write down your deepest thoughts, feelings, or images that show up in these meaningful areas. Try not to worry about the format, just get whatever feels important down on paper as you write for the full 10 minutes. Perhaps see if you can keep the pen on the paper and keep it moving for the full time. If you are unsure what to write, next continue to write the last idea you wrote again and again until maybe something new comes to you.

ADAPTIVE CONDUCT, ETHICS, AND VALUES

As a group, healthy speech, healthy action, and healthy livelihood require an examination of thoughts, deeds, and vocations to determine whether they reflect a motivation that is designed to promote well-being and peace in ourselves and others. Considering ways we might draw upon these practices in serving our patients may require cognitive-behavioral therapists to ponder questions about values and ethics. The Eightfold Path of Buddhist psychology, and in particular the three aspects we've just discussed that deal with adaptive conduct, suggest that the most effective and adaptive thoughts and behavior are *not at all value-neutral*. It suggests that happiness and freedom from suffering are to be found by following a path of virtue—a path defined by compassion, kindness, and the motivation to help not only ourselves but all other beings.

In a sense, training patients in ethical behaviors is somewhat new territory for cognitive-behavioral therapy. However, elements of ethics and values-directed behaviors do emerge in a range of CBT systems. For example, Beckian cognitive therapy and REBT clearly suggest that rationality, positive self-talk, and adopting a realistic perspective are reasonable targets for intervention (Beck, 1976; Ellis, 1962; Laird & Metalsky, 2009). Furthermore, pursuing "experiences of pleasure and mastery" is a part of behavioral activation (Ekers, Richards, & Gilbody, 2008; Jackobson et al., 2001), and "anger management" is a skill that is taught in CBT manuals (Donohue, Tracy, & Gorney, 2009). Despite the nonjudgmental or ethics-neutral stance that CBT clinicians may consciously aspire toward, ethics and values do find their place throughout CBT. In many ways, the nonjudgment that therapists embody has much more to do with being noncondemning of a person's basic humanity. In an adult-to-adult relationship, using both guided discovery and problem solving, both the CBT patient and the therapist are regularly using their judgment to move toward healthier behaviors in most cases.

Values have been defined as "freely chosen, verbally constructed consequences of ongoing, dynamic, evolving patterns of activity, which establish predominant reinforcers for that activity that are intrinsic in engagement in the valued behavioral pattern itself" (Wilson & DuFrene, 2008, p. 66). This definition suggests that values-driven therapy does not seek to impose values upon the patient, but aims instead to help the patient achieve liberation from the dominance of his or her learning history, to generate inherently reinforcing, self-perpetuating patterns of behavior that lead to a life of increasing purpose, vitality, and meaning. Values, in this context, are not goals or moral rules, but patterns of action.

In demonstrating what is arguably a more direct relationship between Buddhist ethical aims and variation upon the CBT theme, CFT (Gilbert, 2010b) formulates the cultivation and strengthening of compassionate qualities as a core feature of the therapy. By establishing the primacy of compassion in its theory and method, CFT takes the bold step of directly suggesting an ethical imperative for practitioners and patients. There is a growing empirical basis for taking this stance, as building evidence suggests that the cultivation of qualities such as loving-kindness (the kind wish that oneself and others be happy) (Frederickson & Cohn, 2008), gratitude (Emmons & McCullough, 2003), and compassion for self and others (Barnard & Curry, 2011; Gilbert & Procter, 2006; Hofmann, Grossman, & Hinton, 2011) can serve to improve happiness, decrease symptoms of psychopathology, and improve well-being. Furthermore, an expanding literature has established that self-compassion is highly correlated with a wide range of positive psychological outcomes, and is negatively correlated with depression, anxiety, and psychological distress (Neff, 2003a, 2003b; Neff, Hseih, & Dejitthirat, 2005; Neff, Rude, & Kirkpatrick, 2007).

Both the Eightfold Path, and the protocols and packages of many of the behavior therapies, may seem to suggest an ethical imperative for human conduct. However, the common ground Buddhist psychology and CBT really share is in establishing and suggesting the development of a particular adaptive set of human behaviors that may lead to the alleviation of human suffering. More than a set of rules, these modalities present us with a map toward effective living, based upon a century of scientific research by psychologists, and two and a half millennia of subjective inquiry by Buddhist practitioners.

4

The Middle Path, Mental Discipline, and Wisdom

Knowledge speaks, but wisdom listens.
—JIMI HENDRIX

The second group of adaptive response patterns that are prescribed by the Eightfold Path involve training the mind, particularly by developing discipline and wisdom in regulating the quality and direction of our attention. We begin by exploring the development of discipline. It has been said that "discipline is knowing what we are able to honourably undertake, and commit to, without any doubt that the undertaking will be discharged with reliability, surety, certainty" (R. Fripp, *www. dgmlive.com*). Cultivating mental discipline in this way involves learning to deploy certain qualities of attention to our moment-by-moment experiences, and to intentionally direct our mental resources toward the alleviation of suffering. Much of what has been imported into CBT from Eastern philosophy explicitly stems from this part of the Middle Path. For example, we can imagine a person with borderline personality disorder who is experiencing an urge to cut himself in response to overwhelming emotions. His habitual behavior in the presence of this emotional suffering has been self-injury. He needs a way to step out of his habitual pattern, and to do that, he needs to be able to harness and direct his attention. Working with attention can be like a spotlight, casting some things into the light, and other things into darkness. Hence, the mental discipline that is involved in a person with such emotion regulation difficulties choosing to engage with a mindful breathing exercise, labeling his emotions, and using his five senses to come into the moment more fully is a clear example of healthy concentration, healthy mindfulness, and repeated healthy effort. The following steps of the Middle Path intervention are a foundation for the effective action many patients need to be able to stimulate.

HEALTHY EFFORT

As with other levels of the Eightfold Path (and like good psychotherapy), we can consider healthy effort in terms of both content and process—what we do and how we do it. Let's start with the "how." The process of healthy effort represents a combination of diligence and inspiration, or as Lama Surya Das puts it, a "skillful balance of endurance, energy, enthusiasm, grace, and dignity" (1997, p. 269). The Buddhist approach recognizes that meaningful life change involves persistent effort over time, inspired by a compassionate and helpful motivation. This persistence is embodied in the methods of Buddhist practice, such as spending years committed to consistent meditation practice or reciting a specific chant or mantra hundreds of thousands of times. In Buddhist psychology, there is a recognition that altering the powerful reflexive tendencies of the mind to grasp and cling takes both time and effort. To endure, this effort needs to be fueled by a powerful motivation: the positive motivation to free oneself and others from suffering.

As for the direction such efforts should take, the Buddha specified four specific pursuits (Das, 1997; Nhat Hahn, 1998; Rahula, 1959/1974):

1. Avoiding engaging in any new unwholesome or unhelpful thoughts or actions.
2. Addressing and working to overcome any existing unwholesome or unhelpful thoughts or actions.
3. Cultivating positive and wholesome states of mind and actions.
4. Maintaining, strengthening, and developing existing wholesome and helpful thoughts or actions.

In maintaining healthy effort, Buddhist practitioners aim to persistently refrain from and address problematic, unwholesome states of mind and behaviors, and to cultivate those that are more wholesome and adaptive, which includes developing our existing strengths. Clearly these efforts map nicely onto the traditional goals of CBT: identifying maladaptive thoughts and behaviors (and the contingencies that maintain them, which Buddhists might call "causes and conditions"), and replacing them with adaptive ones. Like the Buddha, we also are advised to recognize that such efforts require patience, diligent effort over time, and motivating factors that will allow our patients (and ourselves) to sustain these efforts.

The Imaginary Eulogy

The Imaginary Eulogy is an experiential exercise that has many adaptations and variations, and can be found in 12-step work, modern CBT, and contextual CBT (Hayes, Strosahl, & Wilson, 1999, 2011). This values authorship exercise guides the patient through imagining what attending his or her own funeral and hearing his or her eulogy might be like. When we are seeking to stimulate healthy effort, it is important to clearly define and imagine our aim. Beginning with the end in mind, our motivation can be enhanced by having a vivid description of the rewarding, deeply valued consequences that the application of right effort might bring forth. In the following imagery exercise, we are invited to imagine two versions of this eulogy. The first would be the one that we might hear if we were to carry on with our lives with business as usual, without making any major changes in our behavior. The second version of the eulogy represents what we might hear if we were to intentionally live our lives in accordance with our most heartfelt values. This exercise invites patients to ask themselves: "What do I want my life to stand for?" or "What do I want my legacy to be?" This is a guided exercise. It begins with establishing mindfulness or engaging in a brief centering exercises, leads the patient through the guided imagery, and concludes with another brief centering exercise. It may be helpful to have patients write down a few observations when this exercise is complete.

In classical Buddhist practice, there are many meditations on death that can use rather graphic imagery, including the visualization of what happens to the body after we die. Rather than such potentially disturbing, even traumatic, imagery, we have opted to introduce the influence of impermanence on the value of the present moment in a gentler way.

Guided Instructions

As you begin, allow your eyes to close. Begin to focus on your breathing. Settle your awareness on the level of physical sensation, allowing your attention to gather on the breath. Allow each in-breath and each out-breath to flow in its own rhythm. Beyond this, allow yourself to inhabit this awareness, abiding in a state of bare observation, suspending judgment, or evaluation, or even description.

Your mind may wander away from the breath, away from this exercise, and when this happens simply notice the wandering mind and gently return your attention to this practice.

On the next in-breath, begin to imagine that it is 10 years from now and you have won an all-expenses-paid trip to a remote tropical destination. In route, your plane has to make an emergency crash landing and you find yourself stranded. You and your fellow travelers are all safe;, however, you are cut off from civilization. Back home your friends and family are told of the accident and believe that you have died. Unaware of your survival, they begin to plan your funeral. In the mean time, after a week on the island you are saved by a passing fishing boat that unfortunately does not have a working radio. The day you return home happens to be the day of your funeral. You arrive at the funeral moments before your eulogy. Standing at the back of the crowd you go unnoticed and listen as your loved ones speak about your life, what was meaningful to you, about you, what you will be remembered for. As you listen to their words and look around at those who are dear to you. Who is there? Who is speaking? What do they say?

Sit with this experience for a few moments and explore what your loved ones would say if you had continued to live your life including these last 10 years on autopilot, trapped by old habits and struggles with thoughts and emotions, finding yourself on a path that moved you away from what was most important to you.

After spending some time with this, on the next available out-breath, let go of this part of the exercise and with the in-breath gently return your attention to mindful breathing. Noticing the rise and fall of the abdomen as you breathe in and breathe out.

Now, with the next in-breath, begin to imagine that you have arrived at this funeral after having lived your life, and especially the last 10 years embodying your most cherished values and in a manner that reflected your meaning and purpose. Once again, imagine yourself standing at the back of your funeral service, unnoticed and listening as your loved ones speak about you, about your life. As you imagine those people at your funeral, who is in attendance? Imagine yourself watching them listening to your eulogy. And who is speaking? What is he or she saying about those things you said and did? What are they remembering you for?

Allow yourself to sit with this experience for a few moments and consider what your loved ones would say if you had made changes in your life and choices that filled you with purpose and vitality. That you took a path of valued living, engaged with those people, places, and activities that mean the most to you.

After spending some time with this experience, when you are ready and on the next available out-breath, let go of this imagery and with the in-breath gently return your attention to mindful breathing. Noticing the rise and fall of the abdomen as you breathe in and breathe out. Now, with the next in-breath, allow your attention to focus on the sounds that surround you in the room. Next, bring your attention to the sounds outside of the room. Following this, allow your attention to gently settle on the sounds even farther away than that. Giving yourself a few moments to gather your attention and orientation to your presence in your chair, and when you feel ready, you can open your eyes.

Based on similar exercises including a version in Hayes (2005).

HEALTHY MINDFULNESS

Healthy mindfulness is doubtlessly the most widely espoused aspect of the Eightfold Path among 21st-century cognitive-behavioral therapists. Often defined as the kind of awareness that emerges from paying attention to the present moment, on purpose and with acceptance (Kabat-Zinn, 1990), mindfulness involves a flexible and focused attention (Wilson & DuFrene, 2009) that is involved in freeing ourselves from the habitual influences that mental events can bring to our patterns of behavior. The current, widespread use of the term "mindfulness" in CBT is due to the popularization of mindfulness practices in various forms of CBT. In some cases mindfulness has served as a significant component of established treatment models, such as DBT (Linehan, 1993a), ACT (Hayes, Strosahl, & Wilson, 2011), and CFT (Gilbert, 2009a). Other CBT modalities have placed mindfulness as the primary focus of the treatment, as is the case with mindfulness-based stress reduction (MBSR; Kabat-Zinn, 1990), mindfulness-based cognitive therapy (MBCT; Segal, Williams, & Teasdale, 2003), and mindfulness-based relapse prevention (MBRP; Bowen, Chawla, & Marlatt, 2011). In the context of the Eightfold Path, mindfulness refers to being "diligently aware, mindful, and attentive with regards to (1) the activities of the body, (2) sensations or feelings, (3) the activities of the mind, and (4) ideas, thoughts, conceptions, and things" (Rahula, 1959/1974, p. 48). Mindfulness involves the nonjudgmental awareness of whatever is happening in the present moment, awareness that relates to each experience exactly as it is—bodily activities are noticed as bodily activities, feelings are observed as feelings, thoughts and motivations are recognized as thoughts and motivations.

Mindful present-moment awareness, which allows one to recognize thoughts and emotions as activities of the mind, is different from the experience of reality that our patients often inhabit. Clearly, many patients arrive for therapy reporting an experience of reality that is dominated by intrusive and distressing imagery, rumination, and negative emotions driven by harsh and often inaccurate ideas and judgments about the self, the world, and the future (Beck, Rush, Shaw, & Emery, 1979). As a rapidly growing body of psychological literature has shown, training in mindfulness is beneficial in a number of ways, and is associated with improvements in psychological symptomatology, including symptoms of depression and anxiety (Hofmann, Sawyer, Witt, & Oh, 2010) and improved emotional coping (Williams, 2010). Furthermore the study of mindfulness has spawned a large body of neuroimaging research over the last 20 years. As we will discuss more fully in this book, enhanced mindfulness has been demonstrated to correlate with a range of changes in neurophysiological function, and perhaps even neural structure. For example, mindfulness has been associated with significant increases in activation of regions of the brain involved in positive emotions (Greeson, 2009) and increased immune system functioning (Davidson et al., 2003). Some researchers have found that mindfulness training in certain subjects has been correlated with significant increases in the density of gray matter in regions of the brain associated with learning and memory, emotion regulation, the processing of autobiographical information, and the experience of self and perspective taking (Carmody, 2009; Hölzel et al., 2011).

From the vantage point of Buddhist psychology, mindfulness is not just a form of mental training, a mode of attention, or an end in itself. In dharmic terms, mindfulness represents an integral component in a holistic and comprehensive system of promoting psychological and behavioral change in the service of alleviation of suffering.

Mindfulness of the Breath

The use of the breath as an anchor for awareness and the focus of attention is found throughout many different forms of mind training and meditative disciplines. Traditionally in Buddhist psychology, mindfulness of the breath invites us to focus on the ever-present flow of the breath in an open and curious manner. Practices and instructions vary and often begin with discerning long breaths and short breaths, counting breaths, connecting with the experience of the breath, attending to physical sensations of the breath, noticing the effect the breath has on the body, and, finally, using the breath to change the physiological state of the body or relaxing the body. Attention is placed on physical areas of the body that are connected to the sensation of breathing. For instance, the focus may be the entrance or exit points of the breath like the nostrils or back of the throat, or the rise and fall of the abdomen or diaphragm. Some instructions involve using labels such as "in" and "out." Others simply direct attention and awareness to the sensations of breathing such as movement, temperature, or pace. When the practitioner finds that a thought or competing sensation has arisen, he or she is instructed to notice what has happened and where his or her attention has gone and gently return the attention to the experience of breathing with mindful awareness.

Mindfulness of the breath is a central component across the variations of third-wave CBT interventions. Just as DBT practitioners have trained persons with borderline personality disorder to use brief mindfulness-of-the-breath interventions to help them better regulate their emotions, MBCT practitioners have used similar practices as the basis of prevention of depressive relapse and recurrence among patients with chronic depression. In many ways, the practice of mindfulness of the breath is the foundation and wellspring of most of the innovations in third-wave CBT, just as meditation on the breath is the bedrock of Buddhist practice.

In the following mindfulness of the breath practice the clinician is advised to use the written directions to help guide and structure the practice, but to speak from his or her own experience, using his or her own words and pauses when appropriate. This exercise is usually conducted lying down, or seated with the back straight, yet supple. The setting should be at a comfortable temperature, and in a place and time where you will be free from distraction or interruption. As you will find in the guided audio practice available at *www.guilford.com/tirchmaterials*, this practice may be engaged in for about 10 to 15 minutes as one begins to establish a regular engagement with mindfulness.

Guided Instructions

As you begin, allow your eyes to close. Now, gently direct your attention to the sounds around you in the room. If it is quiet, or even silent, just notice the absence of sound, sensing the space around you. When you are ready, after several seconds, bring your attention to the sounds outside of the room. Next, direct your attention to the sounds even farther away than that. On your next inhalation, draw your attention inward to the physical sensations you experience just sitting in this relaxed posture. Just as you did in the mindfulness-of-the-body exercise, allow yourself to collect your attention as you breathe in, observing whatever sensations emerge in your awareness. As you exhale, simply let go of that awareness as the breath leaves the body.

Bring your attention to the presence of life in the lower abdomen. Notice whatever sensations are present as your pattern of inhalation and exhalation continues. Feel the sensations of the abdominal muscles as they expand and contract with the rhythm of your breathing. There is no special rhythm or method with which you should breathe. Allow the breath to find its own pace, essentially allowing it to "breathe itself." With a relaxed, yet attentive, awareness take notice of the changes in sensation as the cycle of the breath continues. As you do this, remain aware that there is no need to change this experience in any way.

Similarly, we are not aiming at creating some special state of relaxation or transcendence. We are merely allowing ourselves to truly be with our experience at this fundamental level, with an attitude of willingness and suspension of judgment, moment by moment. In time, the mind will wander. When this occurs remind yourself that this is the nature of mind, and that this is, indeed, part of the practice of mindfulness. Our mindfulness of the breath exercise involves a cycle of gently returning our attention to the breath, and it is not an experience to be struggled against in any way. When thoughts, images, emotions, or memories arise, we simply allow them to be where they are, making space for them in our awareness. There is no need to fight these mental events off, or to cling to them.

When we notice that our minds have wandered, we simply allow our attention to gently return to the flow of our breathing.

During this entire process, we are intentionally adopting a gentle, compassionate perspective upon the flow of events in our consciousness. As a nonjudgmental and fully accepting observer, we are bringing this quality of kind and patient watching to the river of our mind's activity. From time to time, it may be helpful to ground yourself in the present moment by feeling the physical sensations that you are experiencing. In doing this, you may connect with the sensations of the feet or knees on the ground, your seat on your chair or cushion, your spine, which is straight and supported, and the flow of the breath in and out of the body. You may continue this practice for about 20 minutes before completing the practice. In order to let the exercise go you may again bring your mindful attention to the sounds around you in the room, the sounds that are just outside the room, and the sounds that are farther away even than that. When you are ready, open your eyes, gently rise, and continue with your daily activities.

Based on several sources, notably the guided meditations of Kabat-Zinn (1990). Some of the ideas and phrases are also adapted from the writings of Thich Nat Hahn (1975) and other clinical meditation sources.

HEALTHY CONCENTRATION

The final component of the Eightfold Path dealing with mental discipline is healthy concentration. Healthy concentration involves being able to center and fix attention upon a single point, and to maintain this directed, intentional concentrated attention. Healthy concentration doesn't just refer to maintaining attentional focus. Healthy concentration means being able to bring one's full mental faculties completely to bear on the object of one's attention, free from distraction or tangential thinking. In Tibetan Buddhist practice, it is taught that the process of developing healthy concentration involves moving through various stages. During these successive stages, the ability to maintain a clear, focused, and sustained state of attention progress until even distractingly distressing experiences do not disturb the equanimity and calm of the practitioner. Buddhist psychology and cosmology come together in the formulation and description of such states of consciousness, with the suggestion that, during the experience of deep concentration, the meditator is in more direct contact with the ultimate nature of reality (Nhat Hahn, 1998; Rahula, 1959/1974).

While the tradition of Western psychological science is primarily concerned with objectively observable phenomenon, Buddhist psychology has amassed a wealth of information regarding subjective accounts of the phenomenology of states of deep concentration and meditation. Detailed descriptions of these stages, and instructions for progressing through them, are provided throughout centuries of written accounts of expert meditators. At present many of the central texts of Buddhist psychology have been translated into English. For much of the history of Western psychology, such accounts, and the methods that they stem from, have been largely dismissed. However, the current wave of integration across Western science and Buddhist psychology has begun to take the theory and practice of healthy concentration quite seriously. A founder of the widely respected Mind and Life Institute, the late Francisco Varela, referred to these subjective Buddhist psychology methods as a form of "neurophenomenology" (1997).

While healthy effort, healthy mindfulness, and healthy concentration are described as separate elements of Noble Eightfold Path, we can also see that they are inextricably linked. For example, Zen master Thich Nhat Hahn describes the awareness of mindfulness as providing the foundation for all other aspects of the path, and explains that mindfulness itself requires both diligent effort and engaged concentration (Nhat Hahn, 1998). Practitioners can train all of these capacities within the context of specific individual practices, which may emphasize one element of the Eightfold Path while developing other aspects simultaneously. For instance, the gentle yet persistent self-discipline that is involved in regular mindfulness practice is designed to cultivate diligence, open and vigilant awareness, and increased control over our attention.

Taking the practice of mindful breathing as a case in point, we can notice that a superficially simple practice involves a great deal. As the meditator simply sits with a straight back and dignified posture, he or she fixes a flexible, focused attention upon the flow of breathing. As the mind wanders, the attention is directed, with acceptance and self-compassion, to the breath. This happens many times even in the space of a very brief sitting. The breath serves as an excellent anchor point for developing our attention, as it is always present and easy to find, but subtle enough that it requires more effort than we might expect to keep our attention there. In fact, the entire practice of mindful breathing may be described as an "act of returning." The fact that our minds will occasionally be taken away by thoughts or other distractions gives us the perfect opportunity to practice mindful awareness—learning to notice movement in the mind.

With ongoing practice of mindfulness of the breath, we may begin to notice thoughts and emotions as they initially begin to emerge into our awareness. This last piece is particularly important to attend to when mindfulness is integrated into CBT practice. Some patients may become demoralized when they observe that their minds leave the breath almost as soon as they set it there. As cognitive-behavioral therapists we can see how this observation might set in motion a set of maladaptive cognitions that not only lead the individual to give up on mindful breathing, but to cycle back into immersion in the very patterns of self-criticism and sense of defectiveness that fuel his or her emotional difficulties. For this reason it is important (and accurate) to frame these inevitable lapses in attention as vital opportunities for developing mindful awareness.

When a person is working with weight training for physical fitness, each "rep" that they may do involves pushing against heavy resistance, and then releasing this tension as the weight descends. Without weight and without resistance, the practice would not yield muscle development. The resistance and the motion are essential to the exercise. Similarly, when the mindfulness practitioner engages with their discursive, verbal mind, each distraction is like a single "rep." By engaging healthy effort, healthy mindfulness, and healthy concentration, the "distraction" of the movement of the mind provides the opportunity to gently return to a still point, if even for a moment. All of these capacities are strengthened as they are exercised. Buddhist psychology suggests that we can't learn to notice the emergence of thoughts and emotions in the mind, or to notice when our attention is captured by powerful external stimuli, if these experiences never occur. Practicing mindfulness brings us to a place where choices can be made as to how we engage with our distressing thoughts. From such a place, the range of CBT strategies for behavioral change, self-care, emotion regulation, and alternative cognitive responding can be engaged.

Concentration Meditation: Counting the Breath

In Buddhist meditation, developing and deepening concentration through repeated practice is considered essential. Meditation with an emphasis on concentration is a central feature of *zazen*, the foundational meditation of Zen Buddhism. Counting the breath is an example of an introduction to concentration meditation practice. The act of counting the breath provides a focal point for the mind, and an object on which the mind can sharpen its focus. As has been the case with several of the meditative practices we have described, counting the breath is simple to read about, but more challenging to do. As with any learned behavior, mastery is the result of repeated practice. As such, counting the breath can be helpful when establishing a formal practice. It is recommended to practice regularly and with intention.

In this practice of concentration meditation, the instructions are to count each of your breaths, one at a time, until you reach 10 and then begin again. It is suggested that the counting of breaths be limited to 10 to preserve pointed concentration and prevent habitual counting. When we begin this practice, we will inevitably find that the mind wanders, we have lost our count, or we have become absorbed in some distraction or other. Just as with mindfulness meditation, accepting and making space for such distractions is a part of the value of the exercise. Whenever the mind wanders, simply bring the attention back with the in-breath, and begin the count again. If you reach 10, simply begin again. The counting is done mentally and the simplest instructions are to hold the count or number in your mind for the entire breath. For example, focusing your attention on "one" as you inhale and exhale; then, focusing on "two" as you inhale and then exhale and so on, until you reach 10 and begin counting again with full attention on "one." Again, if you lose track or your mind wanders, mindfully notice that this has occurred and return to counting, beginning again with one. If an open and spacious mindfulness meditation were likened to a wide-angle lens, then we might describe concentration meditation as a zoom lens, where our focus is more guided and directed.

Zen meditation has been integrated into Western psychotherapy by many people since the 1960s. The range of applications has been as wide as mindfulness, though it has not been studied, codified, and disseminated in a similar fashion. One of us (D. T.) developed a concentration and mindfulness meditation-based intervention for PTSD symptoms in heavy combat veterans known as continual awareness training (Tirch & Amodio, 2005). Participants in this group used the focused attention involved in concentration meditation to help them develop an ability to redeploy attention during periods of overwhelming emotion. Mindfulness and open, receiving emotions were used to enhance receptivity to feeling states, while concentration meditation was used to develop distress tolerance. Several participants reported that this ability to modulate the quality of their attention facilitated an ability to successfully deal with being flooded with emotions in preparation for exposure or during challenging situations.

Like the other practices, concentration meditation is typically practiced in a comfortable seated position with a straight back. This meditation is typically completed in silence, so once you have followed the guide a sufficient amount of times to get the feel for the form, you can let go of the audio and practice on your own. Such meditations can be practiced for anywhere from 5 minutes up to 45 minutes. It is a good idea to set a timer, with a soft tone, to alert you to the ending of a period of meditation. Working for a period of roughly 15 to 20 minutes for concentration meditation should provide a workable and thorough daily practice interval. Of course, allow your wisdom to be your guide and explore the edges of your limits with care and patience.

Guided Instructions

As you begin, let your eyes close, and fall still. Allow yourself to gently direct your attention to the physical sensations you are experiencing in the present moment, bringing your attention to the body. In this moment, direct your attention to the flow of the breath, as it moves gently in and out of the body. There is no need to breathe in any special way, just allow the breath to find its own rhythm in time. You may wish to imagine the breath as it descends into the abdomen, breathing fully into the body. See if you can notice the point just below your navel, where your center of gravity rests. Feel the breath resting in this stillness, even as it flows in and out in a steady and slow rhythm. When you are ready, on the next available in-breath, bring your focus to counting, holding each count in your mind—"one," breathing in, and breathing out,—"two," breathing in, breathing out.

Continue counting in this manner and when a distraction arises simply and gently guide your awareness back to the breath, focusing on beginning again with one. So if there is a distraction, then with the next in-breath, begin the count again, "one," breathing in, and breathing out, "two," breathing in and breathing out. Holding each count in your mind with a relaxed yet attuned awareness, a one-pointed concentration for the entirety of each breath.

After you have spent some time attending to the counting of the breath, perhaps 15 minutes, and having brought a mindful awareness to the breath and concentration to the act of counting, over the course of several minutes gently let go of counting and allow your attention to rest on the subtle physical sensations in the breath and body. Giving yourself a few moments to gather your attention and orientation to your presence on your chair or cushion, you can open your eyes, and if you like, acknowledge to yourself the completion of this practice.

THE MIDDLE PATH: WISDOM

The two components of the Eightfold Path that have been grouped together as the central elements of wisdom, healthy understanding and healthy intentions, are often listed as the first and second aspects of the Buddhist system. In a context of comprehensive *dharma* study, this is a logical sequence, as both of these elements directly involve deepening one's knowledge of the broader corpus of Buddhist philosophy. In the context of the integration of Buddhist psychology and CBT, healthy understanding and healthy intentions are more logically sequenced following a description of the practical, overt and covert behavioral dimensions of the Middle Path intervention. As the aims of CBT involve a clinical application of psychological science, pragmatic applications of Buddhist psychology are of more immediate interest than philosophical or ontological assertions. Despite the ongoing integration of mindfulness, acceptance, and compassion into the mainstream of CBT practice, the foundational elements of Buddhist cosmology, philosophy of self, and the degree of interdependence of all phenomena are considerably different from typical Western models. Still, Buddhist models of wisdom, and understanding the essential nature of our universe, do provide opportunities for the CBT practitioner. As such, we are presenting these new, Buddhist psychology models in more familiar forms. We don't wish to describe these concepts as axiomatic teachings or spiritual claims, but as perspectives and insights into what we may come to know of the nature of being, through engagement with contemplative practice, mindfulness, acceptance, and compassion, in our present moment experience. All of this is in the service of the alleviation of human suffering.

Healthy Intention

At the most basic level, we might consider healthy intention as choosing to cultivate an adaptive relationship to our thinking, one that serves the Buddhist aim of liberation from suffering. Accordingly, such a relationship will be resonant with many of the subtler aspects of Buddhist philosophy elaborated in this book. According to the teachings of the *dharma*, thinking in a more adaptive way and having a wise and rational relationship to mental events tends to weaken our obsession with the conceptualized self, and can strengthen an attitude of love, compassion, and nonviolence to all beings (Rahula, 1959/1974). Healthy intention also includes cultivating thoughts that encourage us to diligently work to improve ourselves, and transition our consciousness from a preoccupation with the push and pull of neurotic craving and compulsive avoidance. Buddhist psychology's conceptualization of healthy intention is inherently emotionally validating, insofar as Buddhist psychology recognizes that changing established patterns of behavior and cognition can be quite difficult, particularly given the inevitably challenging circumstances that life presents to us. The cultivation of healthy intention takes into account that modifying deeply entrenched habits of mind requires consistent effort, sometimes over very lengthy periods of time. Relatedly, Buddhist practice incorporates numerous practices that are specifically designed to strengthen one's motivation and diligence to continue practicing, often by cultivating specific patterns of thought. In this way, healthy intention is related to healthy effort.

The various schools of Tibetan Buddhism, for example, encourage practitioners to engage in preliminary practices, or *ngondro*, which are designed to instruct students in how to enter into deeper Buddhist practice and study. Preliminary practices are meant to strengthen a practitioner's motivation, and to prepare the mind for the practices that lie ahead. Some of these preliminary exercises involve the student engaging in specific, repetitive activities, for example, reciting mantras as many as 100,000 times over a period of study. Such chanting involves breathing exercises, mindfulness, and sometimes imagery, or even physical exercise. Extensive, rigorous practice such as this serves many purposes. Cultivation of self-regulation and personal discipline, behavioral activation, and exposure to affect are all CBT processes that may be activated through such activities. From a behavioral perspective, the identification of a specific goal (like 100,000 mantra repetitions) is particularly skillful, because it gives the student a measurable unit of progress toward a goal, increasing motivation along the way and helping to create a tangible referent for what is essentially a rather amorphous process (mental change). Such practices also consider ways to keep the student engaged in the process, because they aren't likely to impact the mind if the student simply thoughtlessly goes through the motions.

Leaves on a Stream

This experiential exercise is an imagery practice intended to increase awareness of thoughts and feelings without excessive attachment or being dominated by the flow of ideas, emotions, and impulses that move through our minds (Hayes, 2006; Hayes, Strosahl, & Wilson, 1999). In this way, a person may be able to better liberate him- or herself from the habitual, narrow range of behaviors he or she might have when he or she is faced with feelings of neurotic craving, aversion, or distorted and overly self-focused thoughts. This practice involves imagining thoughts on leaves or in bubbles as they float downstream. The aim is to use this imagery to practice simply noticing one's stream of conscious experience as it unfolds in an open and accepting manner. This is an imagery exercise that can be guided in session or practiced independently. It begins with establishing mindfulness or engaging in a brief centering exercises, then we engage in the imagery practice, and concludes with another brief centering exercise.

The practice is adapted from ACT (Hayes, Strosahl, & Wilson, 2012), but it has its antecedents in hundreds of Buddhist teaching tales and visualizations. In such culturally situated exercises, Buddhist practitioners may visualize their thoughts or self-conception in many ways. For example, a person may imagine his or her consciousness as a dewdrop, which, upon entering the ocean, dissolves the illusion of a separate self. It is said that as a dewdrop enters the ocean, so the ocean enters the dewdrop. The Leaves on a Stream practice is an example of the applied mindfulness that can facilitate healthy intention, and dis-identification with the flow of our cognitions and emotions. Like many of these exercises, this exercise can be used transdiagnostically with any patients who may benefit from increasing their capacity for decentering, defusion, and mindfulness. There are no particular admonitions or warnings about specific populations that shouldn't engage in this practice to be found in the literature. However, clinicians should be guided by their judgment and case conceptualization in how this practice is applied and with which clients.

Guided Instructions

Find a comfortable position in your chair or on your cushion, adopting a straight spine, and creating a comfortable posture with your hands resting in your lap. As you begin, let your eyes close, and fall still. Allow yourself to gently direct your attention to the physical sensations of your breath in this moment. Simply let yourself observe the flow of the breath, as it is.

When you are ready, bring to mind an image of a slow-moving brook or stream. You may notice the setting surrounding this stream; perhaps it is meandering down a grassy hill, or traveling through a valley of wildflowers. Maybe it is nestled in a quiet wooded area or surrounded by tall grasses and willow trees. As you imagine this stream, notice the water moving over and around green moss-covered rocks and tree roots. Floating on this stream are bubbles, leaves, or wildflower petals that have found their way to the water and are gently carried downstream.

Now, allow yourself to imagine you are sitting on the bank of this stream underneath a tree or among the wildflowers on a warm sunny day as you watch leaves and bubbles float by. While you are imagining sitting by this stream you may notice that your mind has wandered to other thoughts. When this happens, see if you can imagine these thoughts written on one of those leaves or petals as they float by on the stream. If the thought is in words, imagine it as words on the leaf. Or if it is an image, imagine it on a leaf as an image. Simply stay beside the stream and allow the leaves to float down stream at their own pace. If you find yourself swept downstream with a thought, just notice what has happened and return your attention to sitting on the bank of the stream, watching the water and leaves floating by. The same goes for other distractions, if you notice any distractions, feelings, or sensations that arise, picture them on a leaf floating on the water, moving downstream. If it shows up again, simply repeat. Notice its appearance on a leaf and let it float by.

After you have spent some time engaged in this practice and when you are ready, gently allow your breath and attention to settle on the physical sensations in the abdomen. Now, with the next in-breath, allow your attention to focus on the sounds that surround you in the room. Next, bring the attention to the sounds outside of the room. Following this, allow your attention to gently settle on the sounds even farther away than that. Giving yourself a few moments to gather your attention and orientation to your presence on the mat, you can open your eyes, and resume your daily activities.

Adapted from Hayes (2005). Used with permission from New Harbinger Publications, Inc. Copyright 2005 by Steven C. Hayes with Spencer Smith.

Healthy Understanding

Healthy understanding, also called Right View, involves developing a deep understanding of the principles of Buddhist theory, and gaining increasing insight into the underlying psychological processes delineated in the teachings of the Buddha (Nhat Hahn, 1998). It also involves learning to relate to the world directly and objectively, seeing things exactly as they are, unobscured by our fantasies, biases, and deluded ideas (Das, 1997; Nhat Hahn, 1998).

As we consider healthy understanding, it is worth noting that there is a great deal of commonality between Buddhist psychology and CBT in terms of their central observations about the dynamics of emotional disturbances. Both traditions take the perspective that many of our difficulties occur because we tend to respond to mental events as though they were literally occurring in the world around us. CBT and Buddhist psychology also concur in their emphasis on an individual's being served well through a process of learning how to overcome maladaptive patterns of experiential avoidance, or addictive/compulsive behaviors. Such behaviors may be based upon a dominant stimulus function of "craving" being exerted by both internal and external stimuli. This is to say that both Buddhist psychology and CBT agree that when we struggle to avoid the unavoidable, or to attain that which is unattainable or unsustainable, such as euphoric or dissociative "chilled out" states of mind and body, our suffering increases. To accept what we must, and change what we can, in the direction of mindfulness, acceptance, and compassion, is a road to happiness that is shared by both schools of thought.

Buddhist psychology and CBT perspectives alike formulate human suffering as involving reflexive cognition that is considered dysfunctional. This means that such thinking is not functioning to best serve the maintenance of individual or collective well-being. Negative automatic thinking is addressed, in form and in function, by a number of methods in Buddhism and the cognitive and behavioral therapies. Both schools of thought point to the negative impact of our flawed conceptualizations of ourselves, others, and the world as the underlying basis of many of our difficulties.

For example, cognitive therapists may seek to use a process of guided discovery to help patients identify and modify maladaptive negative thoughts. Relatedly, ACT therapists may use perspective-taking exercises to help patients change the narrowing influence that intrusive thoughts have upon their pursuit of meaningful, rewarding lives. Buddhism extends the disruption of the form and function of maladaptive thinking to our most fundamental assumptions about what it means to be a living human being, and what the nature of reality itself may be.

The teachings of generations of Buddhist practitioners and scholars suggest that "things are not as they seem," and that many of our difficulties stem from imbuing our perception of reality with a solidity, a permanence, and an objectively existential status that the universe itself, as we experience it, may not inherently possess. In a context of impermanence, knowing that all that we perceive is the mental mirror of whatever may exist objectively, we continue to reify and concertize our version of how things are, driven by neurotic craving and desperate fears. To the Buddhist, this is the crux of the problem: that the very objects we tend to pursue in attempting to gain an illusory form of happiness are incapable of providing sustained well-being. As the ancient saying goes, "painted cakes do not satisfy hunger." Our struggle and dissatisfaction in life involves our relating to ephemeral representations of the world in a way that grants mental events a level of existence, again a solidity, that they simply do not have. Recognizing, understanding, and ultimately realizing this is Right Understanding.

FROM FOUR TRUTHS AND EIGHT STEPS TO PERSONAL TRANSFORMATION

The Four Noble Truths and the Eightfold Path provide us with more than the foundation of Buddhist psychology. In and of themselves, without religious assumptions, ontological claims, or ritualistic pleas to an interventionist deity, these philosophical observations and practical guidelines for intervention provide an empirically testable program for addressing the problem of human suffering (Dalai Lama, 1991). At this point in the history of the cross-cultural science of the mind and mental well-being, an integration of Buddhist psychology and CBT is accelerating (Keng, Smoski, & Robins, 2011; Ost, 2008; Wallace, 2003). As we step toward this aim, we begin a necessary inquiry into the philosophical, practical, and historical fundamentals of both Buddhism and cognitive and behavioral therapies. From these elements, a full appreciation of the question of human suffering and its potential alleviation can also be approached.

5

Mindfulness as a Foundation in Buddhist Psychology and Cognitive-Behavioral Therapy

Always hold fast to the present. Every situation,
indeed every moment, is of infinite value, for it is
the representative of a whole eternity.
—JOHANN WOLFGANG VON GOETHE

Even the casual observer of CBT research and practice can note the significant influence that mindfulness and acceptance-based practices have had upon CBT development over the last 20 years (Roemer & Orsillo, 2009). Despite exponentially expanding scholarship, theoretical publications in the psychological sciences, and a growing body of research that has emerged from neuroscience and medicine, the concept of "mindfulness" often remains vague in its usage and application (Kabat-Zinn, 2009). Over the course of the past several decades, the term "mindfulness" has been used as a placeholder for a variety of practices that are employed in CBT, which are largely derived from the *dharma* (Tirch, 2010).

MINDFULNESS: CONCEPTUALIZATIONS AND DEFINITIONS

Given this state of affairs, a clarification of precisely what is meant by "mindfulness" is useful for CBT practitioners who are exploring

Buddhist concepts. The original Pali (Old Sanskrit) term that has been translated into English as "mindfulness" is *sati*. According to ancient Buddhist texts, *sati* is a state of mind that can be said to involve a blend of present moment-focused attention, accepting awareness, and memory of one's intention (Kabat-Zinn, 2009; Siegel, Germer, & Olendzki, 2009). *Samma-sati* translates as "healthy mindfulness," and is the form of mindful attention described in the Eightfold Path. *Sati* is a fundamental element of the original teachings of the historical Buddha that readily translates to direct mental training.

Numerous Buddhist approaches, particularly within the Theravada (Elder Vehicle) lineage, begin their programs of mental training with meditations and exercises designed to develop mindfulness. The influential Tibetan teacher Chogyam Trungpa (2005, p. 24) described mindfulness as "the method for beginning to relate directly with the mind which was taught by the Lord Buddha." Subsequent Buddhist teachings clearly emphasize techniques, ethical prescriptions, and philosophical perspectives designed to foster the cultivation of compassion. However, these practices emerge from a foundation in the development of *sati*.

Several writers have observed that the translation of *sati* as "mindfulness" has been in dispute in Buddhist circles over the past several decades (Dryden & Still, 2006; Kabat-Zinn, 2009; Siegel et al., 2009). Differing translations have used such terms as "concentration," "bare attention," and "self-possession" (Dryden & Still, 2006). *Sati* also connotes a concept of memory, that is, remembering to be aware of the present moment itself (Kabat-Zinn, 2009). The ancient Greek term *anamnesis*, which means "un-forgetting" or "self-remembering," also relates to this definition of mindfulness (Allen, 1959). Some mental health practitioners may be familiar with the term *anamnesis*, as it was the original term used to describe a psychiatric interview, dating from the 19th century. *Anamnesis* is also the meditative method prescribed by the central Asian mystical religion of Orphism (Voegelin, 1978). Little known today, Orphism was a widely practiced animistic and contemplative spiritual practice throughout the regions between Greece and the Himalyas during the eighth to fifth centuries B.C.E. Perhaps the best known member of the Orphic religion was Socrates (Reale, 1987).

It is telling that the primary technique of the second wave of cognitive and behavioral therapies emphasizes Socratic questioning, while the third wave of cognitive and behavioral therapy emphasizes the meditative practice known as mindfulness. It is highly likely that the quality of attention known as mindfulness was an integral aspect of the cultivation of rationality, balanced perspective taking, wisdom, and compassion that spread throughout the European, Asian, and African continents during the centuries that have come to characterize the emergence of civilization, empathy, and cooperation (Wilson, 2007). While at first blush mindfulness, cognitive restructuring, compassionate mind training, and logical analysis may all seem to be products of *either* Western *or* Eastern psychologies, we can see that, throughout time, across cultures, this discussion regarding differing orientations to our minds is an aspect of our common humanity.

An awareness of these varying perspectives can shed some light on some varying aspects of the phenomenology of mindfulness practice. Nonetheless, it is clear that usage of "mindfulness" as a description of *sati* in English has gained irrevocable traction, and is firmly established. Additionally, a somewhat standard psychological definition of what mindfulness entails has also emerged.

THE WORKING DEFINITION OF MINDFULNESS IN CBT

The English term "mindfulness" entered Western psychological discussion more prominently after Jon Kabat-Zinn popularized its use in two ways. First, in his MBSR program, Kabat-Zinn (2009) used "mindfulness" as an umbrella term for his approach. This was a part of an effort to secularize and implement methods of meditation and mental training that he had found useful in Buddhist practice. As the scientific study of mindfulness practice has grown, spanning outcome research and basic experimental psychological research, and has extended into several scientific disciplines, this more general use of the term "mindfulness" as a catchall reference to Buddhist psychology concepts in a Western medical context has been less prevalent and less significant.

Kabat-Zinn (1990) also famously formulated an operational definition of mindfulness that has become standard in psychological writing and practice: the awareness that arises through paying attention, on purpose, in the present moment, and nonjudgmentally. An alternative, brief variant of this definition that is also in popular usage is "awareness of present experience with acceptance" (Germer et al., 2005, p. 198). Alternately described simply as "flexible, focused attention" (Wilson &

DuFene, 2009), mindfulness involves accessing a mode of paying attention that is different from the mode most human beings typically dwell in during the flow of day-to-day living.

Mindfulness involves cultivating and accessing an intentional mode of awareness that involves a paradoxical dis-identification from the contents of our conscious minds while gently allowing a nonjudgmental, full experience of the present moment (Segal et al., 2012). Over the course of practice, mindfulness meditation can facilitate "breaking through stereotyped perception" (Goleman, 1988, p. 20) to more adaptively, willingly, and thoroughly process the experience of the present moment.

In third-wave behavior therapies and Buddhist practice, this state of mindfulness is cultivated through various systematic methods, typically involving meditation, movement, and yogic exercises. Although such practices are important in mindfulness training, the concept of mindfulness points to a way of being, and a mode of operation of mind and body, that involves more than a skill one learns through exercises (Hayes, 2002a; Kwee, 1990; Tirch & Amodio, 2006). When construed as a distinct mode of experiencing, mindfulness may be understood as a fundamental process involved in the alleviation of suffering (Corrigan, 2004; Fulton & Siegel, 2005; Martin, 1997; Wilson & DuFrene, 2008). As you might expect, beyond simple meditation, cognitive and behavioral therapists have developed an extensive catalogue of methods to induce or promote the quality of attention known as mindfulness, many of which do not have any resemblance to a conventional conceptualization of meditation.

The Body Scan

The practice commonly referred to as the "body scan" can be found in various meditative traditions and in mindfulness-based therapies such as MBSR (Kabat-Zinn, 1990). In many mindfulness traditions, this practice is among the first that is taught. In yoga, a similar exercise, known as *yoga-nidra* or "yogic sleeping," is foundational. The immediacy and salience of physical sensation as a focus for working to cultivate mindfulness are of great value. The body scan involves deliberately and gradually moving mindful awareness throughout the body. The attention is guided to each part of the body in sequence, mindfully attending to whatever sensations are present. The intention is to cultivate awareness of the body without intending to change or alter the state of the body in anyway, just to simply notice and "be with" the body. The experience of our world is often found in physical sensations and changes. For example, intense emotions are often accompanied by changes in our physiology and various sensations. Training in mindfulness of the body and practice of techniques like the body scan allows patients to learn to observe these physical sensations in a new way.

As is the case with mindfulness of the breath practices, the body scan has been used across many diagnoses and with a wide range of populations. It is often used to assist in emotion regulation, to develop adaptive responses to anxiety, and to help patients with addictive and mood disorders. The potential relaxation component of this practice may be helpful in regulating chronic sympathetic overarousal, such as that found in anxiety disorders. However, some clients with anxiety disorders, particularly those clients with panic disorder, may find an increase in their attention to interoceptive experience to be activating. Accordingly, a skilled clinician can be discerning in his or her teaching of the body scan, choosing the client and the stage of his or her therapy wherein this type of skills training and personal development might be most useful. The practice can be trained in session, and clients can generalize their in-session learning through rehearsal and practice on their own.

Guided Instructions

The exercise is usually conducted lying down, or seated with the back straight, yet supple. It is probably best if you find a comfortable space, and lie there on a yoga mat, rug, or blanket. The setting should be at a comfortable temperature, and in a place and time where you will be free from distraction or interruption. As you begin, let your eyes close, and fall still. Allow yourself to gently direct your attention to the physical sensations you are experiencing in the present moment, bringing your attention to the presence of life in the body. For a moment, direct your attention to the sounds around you in the room. Next broaden this sensory experience to take in the sounds just beyond the room. Then allow yourself to observe the sounds even farther away. With the next breath in, bring your attention back to the body and the experience of breathing. Allow yourself to observe the flow of the breath as it moves gently in and out of the body. There is no need to breathe in any special way; just allow the breath to find its own rhythm in time. As you breathe in, notice the physical sensations involved in the inhalation. When you release the breath, allow your attention to flow out with the exhalation. Each in-breath will involve a gathering, a collecting of attention, and each out-breath will involve a process of letting go of that awareness. At this point, gently direct your attention to the physical sensations you are experiencing throughout the body at this moment. With each inhalation, allow your attention to gather at the contact points where your body meets the mat, chair, or cushion that supports you. As you exhale, notice the feeling of heaviness where your body is supported by the ground.

There is no need to aim for any special state during this practice. There is no need to strive to relax, or to "do" anything at all. Your aim in this work is simply to observe what you are experiencing moment by moment. Without judging, analyzing, or even describing your experience, you will now begin to direct your attention to the different parts of the body. As you gather attention at the level of physical sensation, allow yourself to suspend any evaluations and simply deploy a "bare attention" to whatever it is that you observe. With the next inhalation, allow your attention to move to the physical sensations in the abdomen. Notice the various sensations that accompany each in-breath and out-breath. After staying with this experience for a few seconds, bring your attention up from your abdomen, along the length of your left arm, and into the left hand. Allow your attention to spread, as if it were a warm presence radiating down the arm, all the while noticing the presence of life in the body. Merely observe the sensations in the hand. With each in-breath, allow yourself to imagine the breath flowing into the chest and abdomen, and radiating down the left arm into the hand. Your attention will accompany this inhalation, as if you were "breathing in" an awareness of the physical sensations present in the hand. Without changing anything intentionally in the state of the hand, allow yourself to breathe into the sensations in each part of the hand for several seconds. With each exhalation, allow yourself to let go of that awareness. As you do this, allow yourself to notice the thumb . . . the index finger . . . the second finger . . . the ring finger . . . and the pinky. Next breathe in a collected awareness of the sensations in the back of the hand . . . the palm of the hand . . . and the hand as a whole. When you feel that you have completed your gentle observation of the sensations in the left hand, allow your attention to radiate back up the left arm, noticing the presence of life in the lower arm, the bicep, the tricep, and all of the parts of the arm.

With the next inhalation, allow your attention to gather again in the abdomen. Next, allow yourself to bring this attention to the sensations in the right arm and hand, in the same manner that you used with your left. At a comfortable pace, and with an attitude of gentle, nonjudgmental curiosity, direct your attention to each of the areas of the body in turn. Bringing this attention, breathing into the sensations in each foot (and each of the toes); each lower leg, shin, and calf; the pelvic region; the lower back and abdomen; the upper back and shoulders; the neck and the contact point between the head and the spine; the muscles of the face, the forehead, and the scalp.

Allow yourself to take this slowly, and to engage in the exercise with a spirit of patient, accepting curiosity. When you observe discomfort or tension in any part of the body, again allow yourself to breathe into the sensations. As much as you can, attempt to stay with each sensation, merely observing it, being with it moment by moment. It is the nature of our minds to wander, and it is simply the most natural thing for our minds to do. As you engage in this practice, when you notice that your mind has drifted away from the focus on physical sensations, accept that this has happened, allow some room for this experience in your awareness, and gently draw your attention back to the physical sensations with the in-breath. After you have spent some time engaged in this practice, having brought a mindful awareness to the body over the course of several minutes (this practice can range from 15 to 45 or more minutes) gently allow your breath and attention to return to settle on the physical sensations in the abdomen. Now, with the next in-breath, allow your attention to focus on the sounds that surround you in the room. Next, bring the attention to the sounds outside of the room. Following this, allow your attention to gently settle on the sounds even farther away than that. Giving yourself a few moments to gather your attention and orientation to your presence on the mat, you can open your eyes, and resume your daily activities.

Based on several sources, including Leahy, Tirch, and Napolitano (2011) and the guided meditations of Kabat-Zinn (1990). Some of the ideas and phrases are also based on the writings of Thich Nat Hanh and other clinical meditation sources.

AIMS OF MINDFULNESS PRACTICE IN BUDDHIST PSYCHOLOGY AND CBT

As the Buddhist scholar B. Allan Wallace has noted, throughout Buddhist history, mindfulness training was not pursued as an aim in and of itself. Mindfulness training was a part of the larger scope of Buddhist psychology techniques, and was engaged in as a precursor to the development of further "wholesome states of mind" (Wallace, 2011). According to Buddhist teachings, and current research, mindfulness training cultivates certain capacities of the mind (e.g., attention, awareness, intention, objectivity) that are useful in the subsequent development of wisdom, compassion, and movement toward healthy action (Mosig, 1989).

In addition to the definitions we have explored, mindfulness can also be translated as "to see with discernment" (Shapiro, Astin, Bishop, & Cordova, 2005, p. 165). This discernment applies to all things, internal or external, that are observable by the human mind. Mindfulness is experienced and practiced in order to provide insight and understanding into the true nature of ourselves and the world around us. This is pursued to help create the foundation for cultivating wisdom, compassion, and meaningful transformation (Dalai Lama & Ekman, 2008). Buddhist psychology suggests that to the degree to which our habitual perceptions of ourselves, the world, and others involves egocentric distortion and delusion, we are likely to experience a lack of acceptance and a state of suffering (Germer, 2005a; Olendzki, 2005). According to Buddhist psychology, the attachment individuals have to their consciousness, their view of self and others, and their perceptions of reality is responsible for human suffering (DelMonte, 1995; Hirst, 2003).

Of course, the notion that distorted, dysfunctional automatic thoughts and beliefs drive psychological suffering will sound familiar to CBT practitioners. This central premise is shared with Beckian cognitive therapy, which formulates depression as a negative information-processing bias (Beck & Clark, 1988; Lim & Kim, 2005; Mogg, Bradley, Williams, & Mathews, 1993). Like the Beckian cognitive processes of distancing and cognitive restructuring, mindfulness practice seeks to provide a technique for letting go of attachment to dysfunctional beliefs. Buddhist psychology aims to disregard or question mental distortions that cause suffering by providing a clearer understanding of reality using mindfulness as a context in which this can take place (Fulton & Siegel, 2005; Kabat-Zinn, 2003; Nhat Hanh, 1975; Tirch, 2010).

THE THREE MARKS OF EXISTENCE

While it may seem hyperbolic for the CBT practitioner, from the perspective of Buddhist psychology, mindfulness practice is viewed as the key to unlocking the full potential of the human species (Didonna, 2009a; Kabat-Zinn, 2009). More specifically, mindfulness meditation is designed to deepen the practitioner's understanding of the true nature of his or her existence (Das, 1997). Buddhist psychology operationalizes three aspects of existence, which can be encountered and clarified through mindfulness practice. Known as the Three Marks of Existence, or the Three Dharma Seals (Nhat Hanh, 1973), these aspects of being human are impermanence, no-self, and suffering.

Impermanence

The First Mark of Existence, impermanence (*anicca*, Pali) represents an awareness that all phenomena that we may experience exists in a state of fluid, perpetual change, and eventually will come to an end. Western science has demonstrated that the fabric of our perceived reality consists of vibrations of energy, in a state of motion and transformation at the subtlest level (Dalai Lama, 2011). On a significantly more observable level, we know that all things are in motion in space and in time. Each one of us will eventually die, and that extends to all living things, and even to planets and stars. Ultimately, everything observable, including feelings, figures, perceptions, urges, intentions, and consciousness are interrelated and void of any permanent self-existing or self-defining characteristics (Kabat-Zinn, 2005). When we create a fixed understanding of things, the mind believes that the object of awareness is apparent to others, is permanent, and can exist without the mind that originally perceived or created it (Hirst, 2003). In Buddhist psychology suffering results from this misunderstanding of reality, when an individual mistakes a progression of conditional patterns in constant unrest or change for an enduring entity (Olendzki, 2005). These mistaken views are at the core of how we interpret and shape our existence and experiences in this world (Kabat-Zinn, 2005; Olendski, 2005). This delusion can lead to other dysfunctional, habitual behaviors that are also causes of suffering, such as greed and hatred and attempts to avoid all pain and seek out only pleasure (Epstein, 1995; Surrey, 2005).

As an object of mindfulness, impermanence is experienced beyond conceptual understanding and is considered a practice in service of the clear understanding of reality (Nhat Hanh, 1973). The aim is to develop an understanding that nothing is fixed, permanent, or enduring. This means that everything around us, including the self, is constantly moving, developing, changing and/or evolving (Olendzki, 2005). Mindfulness of impermanence provides the opportunity to appreciate the uniqueness and preciousness of the moment and all that is available to us right now. Impermanence through the lens of mindfulness reveals its value and allows for the letting go of attachment to fixed concepts, objects, and feelings.

This has long been emphasized in CBT. The fact that thoughts, feelings, and moods come and go, that the more we cling to an erroneous belief in how things "should be" or "definitely are," the more likely we are to continue to be met with disappointment when they inevitably change or violate our rules for the universe (Hofmann, 2012). Again, we know that everything that is alive will die. Everything that is young or new will become old or banal. Often, the less we are aware of this reality, the more we tend to suffer or deny ourselves joy or pleasure. Pleasure is innately fleeting, "it cannot be sustained forever, we find, and its completion returns us to a state of impoverishment, of unrest, of separateness, desire, or tension" (Epstein, 1995, p. 26). According to this view, mindfulness allows individuals to see past their perceptions and let go of attachment to public or private events and experience life without needless craving, attachment, or despair (Germer, 2005a; Nhat Hanh, 1973). Being present and experiencing impermanence also gives us insight into the interdependent nature of all reality.

Mindfulness of Impermanence

The only constant is change.
—HERACLITUS

Impermanence is more than an idea, it is a practice to help us touch reality.
—THÍCH NÁHT HẠNH (1998, p. 131)

The illusion of permanence and our attempts to cling to and fuse with our world and experiences is the source of suffering and dissatisfaction. In Buddhism, impermanence means continuous unending change, or transitoriness. The wisdom of impermanence is gained not just through understanding but also through felt experience (Sears, Tirch, & Denton, 2011). Meditations on impermanence aim to cultivate such an experience and deepen the understanding that things

are both interdependent and ephemeral. Additionally, mediations on impermanence address the issue of attachment as a source of suffering. If one has a
wisdom and insight into the impermanent nature of things, then he or she is less
likely to cling to or become attached to physical or psychological experiences or
to physical experiences and those people, places, and things he or she encounters (Bien, 2010). They are less likely to feed false imaginings (*viklapa*, Pali)
"and suddenly they set up barriers between themselves" (Nhat Hanh, 1998,
p. 154). Insight and experiential learning regarding impermanence can lead to
increased psychological flexibility and also lead to behavioral activation toward
valued goals.

Meditations on impermanence range from macro to micro or from gross
to subtle: impermanence exists from a visible, tangible level to a microscopic,
almost invisible level; from the internal to the external environment (McDonald &
Courtin, 2005). Reflections on these different levels of impermanence are important, interrelated, and are found in various meditative practices. On the most
macro level, everything decays, ends, dies. All living beings are in the process
of changing, growing, decaying, and ultimately dying. On the other end, each
moment for each cell and even each atom is always different and changing with
the passage of time. All of our experience is made up of moments, each different
from the last.

Guided Instructions

As you begin, allow your eyes to close. Now gently direct your attention to the
sounds around you in the room. When you are ready, after several seconds,
bring your attention to the sounds outside of the room. Next, direct your attention to the sounds even farther away than that. On the next inhalation, allow
your attention to gently gather at the level of physical sensation. When you are
ready, bring your awareness to the movement of the breath in the abdomen.
Observe whatever sensations are present in the abdomen, allowing your attention to collect and gather on the inhalation, and letting go of the awareness of
particular sensations as you exhale. Allow this breath to flow in its own rhythm.
Beyond this, allow yourself to settle into this awareness, abiding in a state of
bare observation, suspending judgment, evaluation, or even description. It is the
nature of our minds to wander and drift away from the breath. When we notice
this drift of attention, we may even briefly acknowledge ourselves for having a
moment of self-awareness, and gently return our attention to the flow of the
breath. Pay particular attention to your exhalation, noticing the point when the
breath gives way to cessation and to silence. The breath is impermanent, it cannot continue further.

Now slowly begin to expand your awareness of the quality of your breath.
Allow your curiosity to focus on your breath. Is it long or short breaths? What
does the beginning of the breath feel like? The middle? The end? And the beginning of the next breath, what does that feel like? Continue to explore the nuances
of your breath in this way, simply noticing the different or changing qualities of
each breath. It is the nature of our minds to wander and drift away from the
breath. When this happens, make note of where your mind has drifted, briefly

acknowledge the nature of the distraction, and return your attention to the sensation of breathing.

With the next inhale, gradually expand your awareness to include your physical surroundings: imagine yourself sitting on your chair or cushion, the floor underneath you, the space and objects around you, the furniture, the art on the walls, the walls themselves, the ceiling above you. Allow yourself to ponder the physical nature of these things. While they may seem solid, all of these things are made up of small moving particles, energy moving around to cause the illusion of constancy. All is in a state of flux and all is changing, completing and beginning. Allow your awareness and curiosity to stay with this experience, simply noticing the subtle impermanence of life, the true nature of your surroundings.

Now, while attending to this awareness of impermanence, allow this attention to expand to the whole of the building you are in, the plants, concrete, animals, and people in your neighborhood, in your city. You can expand this awareness to the whole of your country, continent, and the earth itself, go as far as you like. Remember that each element, being, and object you include in this awareness is changing and moving in this very instant, always different in each passing moment.

While you allow your awareness to reside in the feeling of the constant change inherent in all things, as best you can, keep your attention on this experience, expanding into and out from this felt understanding. When this fades, begin again, considering the impermanent nature of your breath, thoughts, body, mind, or other object in your awareness.

Before letting go of this part of the meditation, consider the unhelpful tendency we have as human beings to cling to things as though they were solid and constant.

After spending some time with this exercise, on the next out-breath, let go of this awareness and bring your attention to the movement of the breath in the abdomen. Observe whatever sensations are present in the abdomen, allowing your attention to collect and gather on the inhalation, and letting go of the awareness of particular sensations as you exhale. Allow this breath to flow in its own rhythm. Recall the experience of noticing the breath at the beginning of this practice. What is different now? What has changed? Are there sensations that have arisen that weren't there before? Have other sensations changed or dissipated? Spend a few moments noticing the unique qualities of the breath and body in this moment. After practicing this attention for a few minutes, allow yourself to notice when you are ready to bring this practice to a close. Then exhale and to let go of this exercise entirely. At your own pace, bring your awareness back into your surrounding and open your eyes, returning to your experience right now.

Based on exercises in Sears, Tirch, and Denton (2011), McDonald and Courtin (2005), and other sources.

No-Self

The concept of the self in Buddhist psychology is different from common Western conceptualizations of the self. According to Buddhist psychology, the self is an experience that human beings have as a result of the conditioned factors of their existence. This self is not a fixed entity, but a fluid process that emerges from the interaction of a sentient being and its environment. Mindfulness training is designed to facilitate an experience of self that foregrounds these aspects of being. Essentially, mindfulness is meant to facilitate a shift in the experience of the self away from identification with a narrative sense of self and toward an experience of the self as an ongoing process of present moment-focused experiencing. This shift in the sense of self is a hallmark of the phenomenology of mindfulness practice (Mosig, 1989; Nhat Hanh, 1975). It is possible that the apperception of impermanence that arises in states of mindful awareness when focused inward may directly and inherently reveal an experience of *anatta* (Pali). Accordingly, the reverse is also apparent. When we engage in mindfulness of no-self, impermanence may be revealed (Nhat Hanh, 1973). The doctrine of *anatta* implies that nothing has a separate "self" because all beings exist in a constant connection with everything else. Buddhist psychology is grounded in the observation that all phenomena emerge through their direct physical connection with the living universe of which they are intimately a part of (Yeshe & Ribush, 2000). This means that you are more than who you think you are, and "you" are made up of elements that are literally "not you" (Nhat Hanh, 1973).

Most forms of CBT limit the scope of their claims and their scientific focus of convenience to human cognition and behavior. As a prescientific philosophy that sought to pierce the mysteries of being itself, the *dharma* has not subjected itself to such limitations in scope of analysis and inquiry. Nevertheless, *anatta*, in principle, is similar to the popular CBT notion that *we are not our thoughts, we are not our behaviors, and we are not our emotions* (Leahy & Rego, 2012). As we will increasingly examine throughout this text, it is possible that our selves are not as concrete as we often perceive them to be. As the Buddhist psychotherapist Mark Epstein (1995) observes, "Just as modern physics has shown that the observer inevitably distorts that which is observed, so too, we, as experiencing subjects can never know yourself satisfactorily as object. We cannot experience ourselves indivisibly but must experience ourselves as either subject or object, as knower or that which is known" (p. 55).

Mindfulness of *anatta* also provides a practice to help get in touch with the nature of reality and to let go of the distorted labels and stories our mind tells us about ourselves, where we have been, and where we are going.

Suffering

Our earlier description of the various dimensions of *dukkha* in terms of the First Noble Truth only begins to describe what mindfulness of suffering may reveal to us about the nature of our humanity. In mindfulness practice, we do not turn away from suffering, but rather bring our experience of emotional pain, longing, and the unsettling uncertainty of life into close focus and intimate contact. As we have seen, the Buddhist psychology concept of *dukkha*, or suffering, may be better translated as "pervasive unsatisfactoriness" stemming from physical and mental anguish (i.e., old age, sickness, and death); wanting, desire, attachments; and self-dissatisfaction (Teasdale & Chaskalson, 2011). In essence, the Third Mark of Existence is the human capacity for great suffering, met with clear seeing and acceptance, that can resolve itself as an experience of freedom from the behavioral constriction and repertoire-narrowing stimulus functions. Perhaps this is something of what is meant by the notion of "true enlightenment." Paradoxically, in Buddhist psychology, it appears that "causes of suffering are also the means of relief" (Epstein, 1995, p. 16). This is to say that the human mind can be both the origin of, and the solution to, human suffering. In essence, you as a human being and all of us have exactly what we need to achieve meaningful change and the transformation of suffering. We may not be able to transform the more challenging external events in our lives, but we can choose to train our capacity to address our inner life with kindness, wisdom, and mindful awareness.

Buddhist psychology asserts that the experience of liberation from suffering, nirvana, is beyond concepts, beyond *dharma*, and yet is within the human capacity, through cultivation of mindfulness. This means that mindfulness can allow an individual to cultivate a mode of perceiving the act of being that is free from the constrictions and limitations of conventional thought, in a sustained way. As such, mindfulness is an integral part of Buddhist psychology's proposed antidote to human suffering, and it is named among the "seven factors of enlightenment" (Cleary, 1994). At this point in the history of cross-cultural psychology we do not need to accept or dismiss assertions of the possibility of enlightenment as articles of faith. Rather, we can frame scientific questions regarding the processes that are involved in the cultivation of mindfulness, as well as the effects and outcomes that follow from regular training in mindfulness.

The research to date suggests that, in part, mindfulness training's effect does involve these Three Marks of Existence: an awareness of the impermanence of phenomena, a shift in our perspective and sense of self, and a shift in our experience of mental suffering (Davis & Hayes, 2011; Hölzel, Lazar, et al., 2011). Buddhist psychology and CBT both suggest that human suffering results from the dominant influence of dysfunctional thinking patterns upon our behavior, attachment to and reification of such patterns, and a stubborn human tendency to experience mental events in a literal way, with mental events affecting our behavior and emotions as though they were events in the outside world (Beck, 1970; Clark, 1996; Dalai Lama, 1991; DeRubeis, Tang, & Beck, 2001). Thus, to achieve meaningful change and relief from suffering, both Buddhist psychology and CBT guide a person to view his or her thoughts concerning the self, the world, and the future in new and psychologically flexible ways. Therefore, by bringing the Three Marks of Existence into mindful awareness, a new perspective and understanding of how our minds function emerges. With this insight, some may experience a deepening of wisdom that will provide guidance toward meaningful change.

THE FOUR FOUNDATIONS OF MINDFULNESS

Mindfulness training in Buddhist psychology has four foundational components, originally known in Pali as the *Satipatthana*. These foundations are elaborated upon in the *Satipatthana Sutta* (Thera, 1998), which essentially translates as the "Teachings of the Foundations of Mindfulness." These teachings suggest four different domains of human experience, which can serve as both the focus and the context for the cultivation of mindfulness, that include:

- *Kaya-sati*: mindfulness of the body
- *Vedana-sati*: mindfulness of feelings
- *Citta-sati*: mindfulness of the mind or consciousness
- *Dhamma-sati*: mindfulness of mental phenomena

In the vast and elaborate body of Buddhist literature concerning the nature of mind in meditation, each of these foundations is addressed in great detail, and is broken down into finely grained descriptions of experience. The CBT clinician may not need to spend time studying these distinctions in great detail. However, experientially learning about each of these foundations provides us with insight into elements of mindfulness that can be subsequently trained. Additionally, descriptions of the Four Foundations teach us about how a Buddhist perspective can highlight subtle aspects of human conscious experience that are not immediately apparent in the literature and taxonomy of Western psychology.

The first foundation of mindfulness is translated as mindfulness of the body or "contemplating the body in the body" (Thera, 1998). In Buddhist psychology traditions, all aspects and processes of the body can be used to develop mindfulness. Classically, mindfulness of the body is about being in direct, conscious contact with the tangible, grounding oneself in both physical form and function. In other words, mindfulness of the body is directed toward pure physical or physiological experience. It is where mindfulness begins.

"Meet your patients where they are" may be one of the first axioms that many new therapists are taught. In a sense, the body is where we are, and where our patients are, in the most direct way. Your body is always here and now, wherever here and now may be. Additionally, your body is always changing. The body is an ongoing example of both gross and subtle aspects of the Three Marks of Existence, in constant states of change.

Like so many things, the body can be both a source of significant suffering and the alleviation of suffering. For example, panic disorder involves an intense, recursive experience of physical symptoms of anxiety that can accelerate into such extreme states of fear and arousal that a person may believe that he or she is dying. Under such conditions, people tend to attempt to avoid or suppress the experience of anxiety, which only serves to amplify and perpetuate the panic attack itself. The most successful forms of CBT for panic attacks involve turning toward the anxious arousal, and directly experiencing the anxious arousal without unnecessary defenses, facilitating habituation (Craske et al., 2010). Buddhist psychology instructions for deploying mindfulness of the body have similar implications. Buddhist practitioners are directed to turn their attention toward their physical experience, while suspending their judgments.

Mindfulness of the body involves a number of aspects, as historically explained. In each of these aspects, the CBT clinician may find a new avenue for intervention, and new possibilities to adapt his or her practice to the needs of a particular patient, truly "meeting the patient where he or she is." For example, many CBT clients find it difficult to label their feelings with words that actually refer to emotions. This tendency toward *alexithymia* can be found in persons with generalized anxiety disorder, borderline personality disorder, and other problems. Often, drawing nonjudgmental attention to physical states can be a doorway to enhancing emotional processing, as in the following brief example of our client Rita.

CLIENT: I was about to enter the office for that job interview and I just felt like I couldn't walk through the door.

THERAPIST: You felt really frozen, huh? What was the emotion that you were feeling?

CLIENT: I don't know. I can't put a word to it. It was just like I wanted to get out of there.

THERAPIST: Great job noticing that action urge. So what did you feel physically? Where did it show up in your body?

CLIENT: My shoulders were tense and I had butterflies in my stomach.

THERAPIST: And what feeling word would you put to that?

CLIENT: I was afraid.

This transition from bodily experience to emotional awareness fits the rubric of Buddhist psychology well, as the second foundation of mindfulness is known as mindfulness of feelings. In this practice feelings are seen as more simplistic, and involve sensory responses to stimuli. This is distinct from more complex, multimodal experiences such as emotions or affect. Traditionally this practice involves noticing your mind as it reacts to experience in either a positive or pleasant ("I like"), negative or unpleasant ("I don't like"), or neutral ("I have no opinion") way. In behaviorist terms, these feelings involve the experience of being under appetitive or aversive control. Mindfulness of feelings involves paying attention to how you experience what is going on right now in a simple, curious manner. This includes the perception of direct sensation. When we practice, we bring bare attention to each feeling tone of our experiences as they arise and fall, resisting the urge to cling to or to avoid the feeling.

There are many ways to practice mindfulness of feeling. Often using the five senses is a good place to start, especially with taste or smell. Our feelings about food and certain odors can be quite clear to us. For example, the smell of fresh baked cookies or spoiled milk elicit strong "like" or "do not like" responses. The key in cultivating mindfulness of feeling, as is the case with all objects of mindfulness, is to work to get unstuck from the habitual patterns of responding that we find ourselves stereotypically locked into from the basis of our learning history. This may be described as "changing our relationship to our feeling states," but we are really talking about a broader freedom. This is a freedom to witness our experience and choose our course of action.

When we discuss the third foundation of mindfulness, mindfulness of mind, we are really discussing a mindfulness of consciousness itself. The original Pali term for consciousness is *citta*, sometimes described as referring to mental events, or the mind itself. However, what the term actually refers to is consciousness, operationalized as an ongoing awareness of internal or external events and changes in our context. Often this event or change is referred to as an object. However, just as the term "stimulus" actually refers to a change in our environment that we perceive rather than an object in our environment itself, the object of consciousness in a real sense involves a change in our relationship to our environment. Similarly, *citta* is an awareness of an "object." The awareness that is referred to as *citta* or consciousness is not the deliberate, cultivated awareness that we encounter in mindfulness. *Citta* refers to everyday, nonintentional awareness. For example, I may have a passing awareness of the object on my desk or the sound of the people walking by just outside my window, without directing purposeful attention toward these events. The *Abhidamma Pitaka* (Bodhi, 2000b), the seminal third century C.E. text that enumerates and systematizes foundational Buddhist thought, establishes that the mind consists of more than what we describe as "consciousness." According to this source, our mind is comprised of a coming together of many elemental components and mental factors such as contact, perception, attention, preference, and many others. In the *Abidhamma* system, 52 constituent mental factors are elaborated, and grouped into three areas; feeling, perception, and mental constructions. In case it hasn't quite hit you yet, archaic Buddhist psychology is often organized by numbered lists of smaller components. When we have a supercomputer built into our handheld phone, it might seem silly to have series of mnemonic devices built into the numbered lists of key points. Anyone who has gotten through graduate school or medical school in the pre-Internet era (perhaps we should call that era B.I.?) can appreciate how chunking complex contests into memorable lists can help us to retain key information. Apparently, Buddhist scholars were early adopters of this kind of method. However we divide and describe the layers and elements of mental activity (and the cognitive and behavioral therapies have many of their own taxonomies), the key in the third foundation of mindfulness is to recognize that we can bring reflexive mindful awareness to our awareness itself.

The fourth foundation of mindfulness refers to a mindfulness of *dhamma*, or mental events. This refers to bringing mindfulness to the contents of consciousness itself rather than observing the process of consciousness. For example, when we bring mindfulness to the experience of a thought, we are practicing the fourth foundation of mindfulness. Metaphorically, if the third foundation of mindfulness were to represent an awareness of a clear blue sky, the fourth foundation would represent our awareness of the clouds, birds, or colors moving through this sky.

In terms of applied Buddhist psychology and CBT, we can see the Four Foundations as a succession of foci for deployed mindful awareness, and also as key interacting processes involved in mindfulness. In Buddhist psychology through working with the Four Foundations of Mindfulness, we learn that we can bring attention to our physical presence in this very moment. We then come into contact with a mindfulness of the urges and embodied emotional sensations that move through this physical, human, embodied intelligence. We learn how to approach these emotional feelings and sensations with willingness and curiosity during our mindfulness practice. From such a point, our awareness can rest, nonjudgmentally, on our spacious, interior landscape of conscious awareness. Rooted in a mindful observation of this field of awareness, we can deploy mindfulness to mental events, experiencing them for what they are. From such a place, we can experience the mental events and internal triggers that habitually guide and often dominate our behavior in maladaptive ways, without surrendering our course of action to them. Hence, the four processes outlined in Buddhist psychology interact to provide us with an opportunity for clear seeing, right action, and the cultivation of healthful states of mind.

The Four Foundations of Mindfulness point to analogous processes in the cognitive and behavioral therapies, in a number of CBT modalities. For example, in the psychological flexibility model, mindfulness is broken down into four core components, which represent behavioral processes that interact to create more adaptive and psychologically flexible functioning (Hayes, Strosahl, & Wilson, 2012). These behavioral components of mindfulness are contacting the present moment, willingness and acceptance of our experience in this moment, inhabiting the perspective of an observing self or self-as-context for mental events, and defusion, or holding our thoughts and emotions more lightly, and getting as free as we can from the habitual influence of our literalized experience of mental phenomenon. All of the psychological flexibility processes involved in mindfulness can be focused on the body, feelings, consciousness, and mental events. Furthermore, these four processes described do not equate to the Four Foundations of Mindfulness, precisely. However, we can use the relationships among these concepts to understand some of the dynamics of mindfulness in Buddhist psychology and CBT.

Using our imagination, and perhaps memory, let's create a scenario in our minds. A person has had some stress and trouble in his or her daily life, and waking to begin a new day. Perhaps he or she struggles with anxiety, and is practicing mindfulness as a part of a CBT program. As part of his or her personal practice, he or she takes his or her seat on a meditation cushion or chair, and begins a mindfulness practice, perhaps a simple mindfulness of the breath exercise. Let us imagine how through the psychological flexibility core process of making "contact with the present moment," he or she brings his or her awareness to the present moment, grounding him- or herself in physical sensation and practicing mindfulness of the body. Deepening his or her morning practice, he or she notices the flow of sensations and emotions, fleeting senses of "like and dislike," or even emotional spikes. Our mindfulness practitioner may bring his or her attention back to the breath, deploying mindfulness of feeling, and practice acceptance and willingness to remain in contact with his or her flow of experience. As he or she stays with the practice, the default mode of mind will arise, and images, thoughts, and fantasies will move through the mind. Practicing mindfulness of consciousness, our meditator is able to recognize that he or she is viewing all of this as a flow of events through an expansive field of awareness. The noticing of the interiority and spaciousness of the mind can be described as bringing awareness to the experience of self-as-context, engaging in flexible perspective taking. As each new mental event and fantasies begins to grip awareness and exert its habitual influence, the mindfulness practitioner engages in defusion, noticing thoughts as thoughts, rather than responding to them as though they were literal events in the world. Hopefully the core processes involved in mindfulness, as described in Buddhist psychology and the behavior therapies, help this client to let go of the suffering and limitations that the craving and avoidant mind can inflict upon him or her. Hopefully our clients can use mindfulness as a foundation for the cultivation of ways to release themselves from needless suffering and live meaningful lives. This aspiration applies to us all, and points the direction that naturally arises from mindfulness practice—the practice of mindfulness as a context for the cultivation of compassion and liberation from suffering.

Mindfulness as a Context for the Cultivation of Compassion

To see one in all and all in one is to break
through the great barrier which narrows one's
perception of reality.
—THÍCH NÁHT HẠNH

As we have observed, cognitive-behavioral therapists have significantly expanded the scope of scientific and cultural influences that inform their research and practice over the past 20 years. As CBT has advanced, it has drawn concepts and techniques from an expanding range of sources, including Buddhist philosophy, new behavioral accounts of language and cognition, and affective neuroscience (Hayes et al., 2004; Kwee, 1990; Mansell, 2008). Increasingly, mindfulness and acceptance-based approaches have come to characterize the public face of innovation in contemporary CBT. A further, more recent trend at the edge of CBT research and development involves compassion-focused approaches, such as CFT (Gilbert, 2005a) and the mindful self-compassion (MSC) program (Neff & Germer, 2013). This emphasis upon compassion within CBT mirrors a greater integration of compassion-focused methods and Buddhist influences within psychotherapy in general (Germer et al., 2005).

Within prescientific Buddhist traditions, mindfulness training is often a beginning point for the novice monk or lay practitioner (Mingyur, 2007). In this context, the practice is seen as serving several purposes. First, it serves as a means to train the powers of attention, so that meditators can eventually focus themselves single-mindedly as they pursue the development of other qualities without the continuous distraction of a wandering mind. From this foundation, the Buddhist student will proceed to learn and practice more advanced methods for cultivating various mental states. One of the primary states that Buddhist practitioners seek to develop is a felt sense of compassion for the self, for others, and ultimately for all beings (Thurman, 1997). This is true in many schools of Buddhist practice, including Theravada, Zen, and Tibetan Buddhism. The sequencing of this mental training would suggest that there is a relationship between the experience of mindfulness and the experience of compassion, wherein mindfulness may serve as a context for compassion-focused approaches.

While mindfulness has been the topic of numerous evolving therapeutic approaches, the emphasis upon the purposeful cultivation of compassion toward oneself and others is a domain that has only recently begun to be explored as the foundation for a therapeutic intervention. This evolving effort will take many forms, both theoretical and empirical. The purpose of this chapter is to explore the potential role of mindfulness as an important and perhaps essential step in the successful cultivation of compassion as more than an affective experience or a fleeting state of mind. An examination of the relevant theoretical, clinical, and neuroimaging literature reveals that both mindful awareness and a felt sense of compassion may be interrelated dimensions of human functioning, having their evolutionary roots in human relational behaviors. Just as an individual Buddhist practitioner may use mindfulness training to prepare his or her mind for the development of compassion, the field of CBT has sufficiently integrated and developed mindfulness-based interventions to prepare a foundation for the use of compassion as an active psychotherapy process. Later chapters will take us deeper into an understanding of compassion in Buddhist psychology and CBT. First, though, in order to examine how mindfulness can provide a foundation and a context for compassion in mental training and in neural expression, we need to familiarize ourselves with the basics of what we mean by "compassion."

AN INTRODUCTION TO CONTEMPORARY CONCEPTUALIZATIONS OF COMPASSION

Compassion-Focused Therapy

Many therapies discuss the value of warmth and empathy in the psycho-therapeutic relationship (Gilbert & Leahy, 2007). However, CFT and other compassion-focused approaches are characterized by an emphasis on the patient's specific training in methods aimed at cultivating a felt sense of compassion for self and others. Compassion-focused approaches hypothesize the cultivation of compassion to be a central process in emotion regulation and in successful therapy, particularly when dealing with patients who struggle with feelings of shame and who exhibit prominent self-critical cognitions (Gilbert & Irons, 2005).

CFT founder Paul Gilbert (2007) describes compassion as a "multi-faceted process" that has evolved from "the care-giver mentality" found in human parental care and child-rearing. In his concise definition, Gilbert (2009a) describes compassion as *a sensitivity to the presence of suffering in self and others with a commitment to try to alleviate and prevent such suffering.* The definition points to two basic aspects of compassion, which are sometimes referred to as the "two psychologies" of compassion by CFT practitioners. The first aspect is *engagement*—involving an opening up to, and a willingness to work with, suffering. The second aspect is *alleviation/prevention*, which involves working to develop the wisdom and skills necessary to alleviate/prevent the suffering. This two-faceted conceptualization is consistent with Buddhist definitions of compassion, which emphasize the combination of a sensitivity to suffering and a motivation to alleviate it.

The psychology of engagement involves identifying and cultivating specific competencies, described as "attributes." These include accessing the motivation to be caring, sensitivity to distress, sympathy, distress tolerance, empathy, and nonjudgment. These qualities of the psychology of engagement are drawn from the research on care-giving behaviors and altruistic behaviors, and they appear to be the foundational elements of a compassionate orientation (Gilbert, 2010a). The psychology of alleviation/prevention involves further competencies for appropriate reflection and action, described in the compassion circle as "skills." CFT uses a systematic approach to train and cultivate these capacities and skills to develop compassion.

The underlying theory for CFT links "psychotherapeutic processes with evolved psychological systems, especially those associated with social behavior" (Gilbert, 2007, p. 109). Drawing from both evolutionary psychology and affective neuroscience, Gilbert distinguishes different affect regulation systems that operate in human beings. Specifically, Gilbert's model involves three systems; among these systems there is a contrast between a threat-focused emotional system, a system that involves emotions based on drives to seek pleasure and acquisition, and a system that focuses on affiliative emotions that involve a felt sense of soothing and safeness (Gilbert, 2005a, 2007, 2009a). The threat-focused system has emerged from older evolutionary structures in the brain, such as the amygdala and the limbic system. It is conceptualized as evolving to favor the activation of sudden and maximally effective defensive behavioral responses, such as the classic "fight, flight, or freeze" responses. In contrast, affiliative-focused behaviors involve an evolved capacity for human beings to feel "safeness" and to feel soothed in the presence of stable, warm, empathic interactions with others (Gilbert, 2009a). This affiliative-focused "safeness system" involves nonverbal behaviors that may resemble the stable, caring context that an engaged and effective parent may establish with his or her child. One of the aims of CFT is to train patients in accessing and employing this system of self-soothing through the felt experience of compassion.

In a similar conceptualization of compassion, Wang (2005) hypothesizes that human compassion emerges from an evolutionarily determined "species-preservative" neurophysiological system. This system is hypothesized as evolving in a relatively recent evolutionary time frame, compared to the older "self-preservative" system. This "species-preservative" system is based on an "inclusive sense of self and promotes awareness of our interconnectedness to others" (Wang, 2005, p. 75). Relative to some other animals, human infants and children may seem defenseless, requiring, as they do, a great deal of care and protection in their early life. As a result, particular brain structures and other elements of the nervous and hormonal systems have evolved to promote nurturing behaviors, which involve protection of and care for others. Basic examples of this evolutionary progression can be observed by contrasting the parenting behaviors of reptiles and amphibians, for example, to that of mammalian species; the former lack even the most basic nurturing behaviors toward their own young, while mammalian species (e.g., rats) can be observed to display a wide range of caretaking behaviors. Moving higher on the evolutionary ladder, Wang's (2005) review of the relevant literature suggests that the human prefrontal cortex, cingulate cortex, and the ventral vagal complex are involved in the activation of this "species-preservative" system. These structures are all involved in the development of healthy attachment bonds, and may also be involved in the cultivation of mindfulness (Siegel, 2007b).

An Introduction to Self-Compassion

In a related approach, Kristin Neff has infused Western social psychology with fundamental elements of Buddhist philosophy to develop a theory of "self-compassion," which is distinct from both "self-esteem" and compassion for others (Neff et al., 2007). According to Neff, self-compassion involves three primary elements: self-kindness, an awareness of our common humanity, and mindful awareness. Neff has developed a self-compassion measure, the Self Compassion Scale (Neff, 2003a). Higher levels of reported self-compassion have been found to be correlated with lower levels of depression and anxiety (Neff, 2003a; Neff et al., 2005; Neff, Kirkpatrick, & Rude, 2007). These relationships have been found to persist, even after controlling for the effect of self-criticism. Neff and colleagues' research has demonstrated positive correlations among self-compassion and a range of positive psychological dimensions (Neff, Rude, & Kirkpatrick, 2007). These factors include, but aren't limited to, life satisfaction, feelings of social connectedness, personal initiative, and positive affect (Neff, Rude, & Kirkpatrick, 2007). As Neff's conceptualization of compassion explicitly involves a Buddhist concept of mindfulness awareness, it represents a bridge between Eastern and Western thought, which is informing an observational and experimental research program.

Finding Compassion in Buddhist Psychology

It is difficult to overstate the importance that compassion plays in most Buddhist traditions. As we have seen, historical accounts characterize the historical teacher who came to be known as "The Buddha," Sidartha Gotama, as a prince who led a privileged and sheltered life that he was moved to abandon upon being exposed to the tremendous suffering of others. This story provides a context for understanding how compassion holds such a revered place in Buddhism. In this way, the very basis of

Buddhism can be attributed to the experience of compassion—with the Buddha experiencing a strong compassionate reaction to the suffering of others (and in the future, himself), and committing the rest of his life to understanding the nature of suffering and learning how to free himself and others from it.

Furthermore, compassion provides the conceptual basis of an entire branch of Buddhism, the Mayahana, which extends the Buddhist goal of achieving enlightenment for oneself to pursuing it for all sentient beings. This perspective is made manifest in the *Bodhisattva* ideal, which will be explored a great deal later. *Bodhisattva* is translated from Sanskrit as "a person whose essence is perfect knowledge." The use of the term *Bodhisattva*, or "awakened being," has changed over time and tradition. Originally, it was used to refer to the historical Buddha prior to his attainment of enlightenment. Later the term came to refer to any individual who is motivated by great compassion and is committed to both learning and teaching effective means of eliminating suffering. In Chinese and Japanese Buddhist mythology, the *Bodhisattva* of Compassion is known as *Guan Yin* or "She Who Hears the Cries of the World" (Collier, 2011). The *Bodhisattva* commits him- or herself entirely to freeing all beings from suffering, with some traditions even suggesting that the *Bodhisattva* delays his or her own pursuit of enlightenment so that he or she can continue to take rebirth in order to continue working to free all beings from suffering. This ideal is described in detail in one of the most cherished texts in Tibetan Buddhism, Shantideva's *A Guide to the Bodhisattva's Way of Life* (Shantideva, 1997).

Several concepts from Buddhist psychology relate to the term "compassion" as it is coming to be used in cognitive and behavioral therapies. The first, and possibly the most directly related, term is *karuna*, which is a Pali term that translates as "compassion" (Rahula, 1959/1974). Specifically, *karuna* involves a desire to prevent harm and suffering from occurring to others and the self. It is a general term, which readily translates to our Western notion of compassion as involving a concern for the prevention of the suffering of others, and it is a quality that is seen as essential in Buddhist teachings.

A second, related Buddhist concept of compassion, *metta*, is usually translated as "loving-kindness." *Metta* involves a desire to bring happiness and positive emotional experience to others, the self, and ultimately, to all sentient beings (Rahula, 1959/1974). *Metta* meditation is perhaps one of the most commonly practiced forms of compassionate mind training in contemporary Western Buddhist practice. During this meditation, the practitioner visualizes him- or herself as an innocent being, and trains him- or herself in the direction of physical, conceptual, and imaginal aspects of compassion toward the self (Kornfield, 1993). It is worth noting that this practice emerges in the *Theravada* tradition, wherein meditation training begins with mindfulness practice, and proceeds to more advanced practices that involve the cultivation of qualities such as *metta*. In this tradition, mindfulness serves as the context for the further development of compassion.

The third Buddhist concept related to the development of compassion is the concept of *bodhicitta*. *Bodhicitta* is a rather more complex concept to grasp for most Westerners, as it involves a Buddhist conceptualization of the self. A Buddhist view of the self stresses an interdependent nature of existence, suggesting that all phenomena are inextricably interwoven. It asserts that the contemplative experience of this great sense of connection will eventually result in an arising altruistic aspiration to work toward the alleviation of suffering for all beings. This arising motivational imperative, known as *bodhicitta* (awakened heart) (Chödrön, 2003), is a major foundation of Buddhist practice.

MINDFULNESS, SOCIAL NEUROPHYSIOLOGY, AND COMPASSION

Human emotion, cognition, awareness, and meta-awareness has emerged through an interaction of evolutionarily derived, genetically transmitted neurophysiology and learned behavioral responses to environmental challenges (Panksepp, 1994). Over the past 20 years, research in mindfulness has moved toward the establishment of models of evolutionary neurophysiology that relate to attachment, compassion, and regions of the brain associated with social functioning. In fact, an evolving body of work points to specific brain areas as being related to (and likely impacted by) both mindfulness practice and the cultivation and experience of compassion. This research has particularly highlighted the role of the insula, the anterior cingulate cortex (ACC), and the middle prefrontal cortex. An exploration of these neurophysiological models will allow us to better understand the role of mindfulness as a context for the further cultivation of compassion.

Based on his work in interpersonal neurobiology and his subjective experience in mindfulness training, Daniel Siegel (2007b) has developed a theory of mindfulness that views mindful awareness as a special relationship with the self, using the brain's social hardware to cultivate an attuned awareness of internal mental processes, which promotes neural integration. The central concept of this perspective is that the quality of focused attention that a caregiver brings to his or her child while fostering healthy attachment bonds, referred to as "attunement," is being brought to the self through mindfulness training. Siegel characterizes the quality of attention in mindful awareness practices as involving "curiosity, openness, acceptance and love (COAL)." Synthesizing the work of other researchers, Siegel's text *The Mindful Brain* (2007b) outlines the ways in which the brain's central hub of social circuitry is involved in, and activated by, mindfulness practice. This perspective is entirely in accord with current research in compassion-focused approaches to therapy, which specifies similar processes and points to similar neural structures (Gilbert, 2005b, 2007, 2009b; Neff, 2009; Wang, 2005).

Research has also suggested that mindfulness training may affect more than regional brain activity, and may actually be associated with structural changes in the brain itself. Sara Lazar and colleagues (2005) conducted neuroimaging research that revealed increased thickness in both the middle prefrontal area and the right insula. This thickening was more pronounced in practitioners who had been practicing mindfulness meditation for a longer period of time. As has been noted, the middle prefrontal areas are often associated with caregiver behavior, and have been suggested to be involved in the experience of compassion (Wang, 2005). The insula serves as a communication channel between the limbic system and the middle prefrontal areas. Information about bodily sensations, emotions, and the representation of others is hypothesized as being linked and synthesized through the action of the insula (Critchley, 2005; Siegel, 2007a, 2007b). Insula functioning has been linked with the experience of compassion, with studies revealing relationships between the level of insula activation and self-reported intensity of compassion-loving-kindness meditation (Lutz, Brefczynski-Lewis, Johnstone, & Davidson, 2008), and with increases in insula activation in response to images of human suffering observed in individuals who had participated in only 2 weeks of *metta* meditation—increases that were positively related both to scores on Dr. Kristin Neff's Self-Compassion Scale and to altruistic behavior (Davidson, 2007, as cited in Germer, 2009). This research is groundbreaking in that it represents structural evidence of "experience-dependent cortical plasticity" associated with meditation training.

In a comprehensive review of electroencephalographic (EEG) and functional magnetic resonance imaging (fMRI) imaging studies of meditation, Cahn and Polich (2006) found that meditation involved increased regional bloodflow to certain areas during the act of meditating. Although Cahn and Polich did not limit their research to mindfulness meditation practices, all of the meditation practices that they studied involved some elements of mindfulness and focused concentration, with varying degrees of emphasis. As a result, their observations concerning brain behavior during meditation are particularly relevant. Overall, meditation appeared to involve changes in the ACC and in dorsolateral prefrontal regions of the brain. Cahn and Polich attribute increased activation in the cingulate cortex and the prefrontal and orbitofrontal cortices found in meditation imaging research to an increase in attentional focus. However, they note that Bartels and Zeki (2004) have also related the functioning of the ACC to the experience of "love." Indeed, researchers have established that the middle prefrontal cortex and the ACC are involved in attachment and caregiving, as well as in attentional and decision-making processes (Siegel, 2007a). Accordingly, here we may note the connection between cultivation of meditative attentional capacities and the emergence of warmth and empathy. CFT seeks to create states of mind that activate specific brain systems such as those linked to empathy (e.g., the insula, the ACC) in order to facilitate new ways of processing difficult emotional memories or emotions. Meditation and mindfulness also activates, stimulates, and develops important brain systems that facilitate new ways to regulate and work with threats and organize our minds.

In a particularly clear study of the role of the ACC in mindfulness practice, fMRI research has demonstrated that adept meditators practicing a mindfulness of breathing exercise exhibit stronger activation in the rostral ACC and dorsal medial prefrontal cortex bilaterally during mindfulness of breathing, when compared to controls (Hölzel et al., 2007). It has been hypothesized that this group difference may be attributed to a more effective processing of distracting events, and may involve more effective processing of emotions. As noted above, the ACC is hypothesized to be involved in attentional control. However, the ACC is also theorized to be involved in the resolution of conflict, emotion regulation, and adaptive responses to changing conditions (Allman,

Hakeem, Erwin, Nimchinsky, & Hof, 2001). The involvement of the rostral ACC, in particular, suggests that an emotion regulation role is taking place during mindfulness practice (Allman et al., 2001).

More specifically, it has been postulated that the ACC plays a role in neural homeostatic mechanisms that regulates an individual's response to distress (Corrigan, 2004). On the basis of this hypothesis, the state of mind that is cultivated during mindfulness training can be viewed as the core mechanism involved in the alleviation of suffering, through various forms of psychotherapy (Corrigan, 2004). Furthermore, the involvement of the ACC reveals the activation of a structure wherein attention, emotional experiencing, and decision making come together. As noted previously, the subjective accounts of long-term Buddhist meditators suggest that advanced mindfulness training facilitates an emergence of a compassionate awareness and a change in the emphasis of the experienced sense of self. Neurophysiological research in this area is beginning to establish neural correlates for such experience.

Neuroimaging research has further explored the neurophysiological changes that may be involved in such a shift in the experienced self. Research using fMRI technology has contrasted the neural correlates involved in a "narrative" mode of self-reference and an "experiential" mode of self-reference (Farb et al., 2007). A "narrative" sense of self roughly corresponds to a conventional Western view of the self as a pervasive and ongoing, separate individual identity enduring across time and situation. The narrative mode of self-reference has been found to be correlated with the medial prefrontal cortex (mPFC), which is involved in maintaining a sense of self across time, comparing one's traits to those of others, and the maintenance of self-knowledge (Farb et al., 2007). The "experiential mode" of self-reference corresponds to the present moment-focused awareness found in mindfulness meditation, and represents the mode of being that has been described as an "Observing Self" (Deikman, 1982). Additionally, this experiential mode of self-reference resembles a relational frame theory concept, the experience of "self as context," which is to say an experience of the self that transcends verbal relational processing frames such as "I–it," "here–there," and "then–now." Essentially, this is an experience of self that is not involved with the processing of an experience of separateness and locality in space and time.

Farb and colleagues' (2007) research examined the neurological activity involved in these modes of self-reference among both experienced meditators and novice participants in an 8-week mindfulness training. Novice meditators exhibited a reduction in the activity of the mPFC while maintaining an experiential focus, which may reflect a reduction in a narrative sense of self-reference. More experienced mindfulness practitioners exhibited stronger reductions in this mPFC activity. Furthermore, the trained participants also exhibited a more right lateralized network of cortical activity including the lateral prefrontal cortex, the viscerosomatic areas, and the inferior parietal lobe. This network of activity appeared to correlate with a phenomenology of an "observing self" and may indicate a more effective mode of processing emotional memories from a mindful stance. Additionally, novice meditators evidenced a stronger coupling between areas of the PFC involved in narrative self-reference (mPFC) and areas that may be involved in the translation of visceral emotional states into conscious feelings (i.e., right insula) (Damasio & Dolan, 1999). More experienced meditators exhibited weaker coupling between these areas, which may reflect a cultivated capacity to disengage the habitual connection between an identified sense of self across time and the processing of emotional memories, yielding the previously described beneficial aspects of the experience of mindfulness and creating space in which the experience of compassion can blossom. Importantly, compassion does not just involve the flexible perspective taking and broader sense of an observing self that is involved with the researched phenomena. As we will explore later, compassion is an evolutionary, emergent human capacity that involves the coming together of human caregiver behaviors and our above discussed facility in meta-awareness. Compassion is a quality of mind that can organize our experience and transform human suffering.

TWO TRUTHS IN MIND AND LIFE

The experience of two discrete states of being, as described by Farb and colleagues (2007), may be seen as phenomenological correlates of the "Two Truths" postulated by Madhyamika Buddhist philosophy (Tirch & Amodio, 2006). According to the Madhyamika teaching of Nagarjuna (second century), reality can be seen from two perspectives. One is the conditioned representation of reality, subjectively constructed in each individual's mind. Essentially, this represents identification with the stories that our minds tell us. Perhaps this sense of reality and sense of self emphasizes the self-preservative processes in the mind and brain. This perspective is known as "Relative Truth." The second perspective is the nature of things as they "are" devoid of perceptual processing and cognitive interpretation, which is neither objective nor subjective. From this perspective, our sense of self may be connected to our direct experience of being, connected with the environment we coexist with and within. Such a perspective may be more involved with species-preservative mental and neural processes. This perspective is known as "Absolute Truth" in the Madhyamika philosophy. While we may experience ourselves as separate beings with a consistent sense of self, Buddhist philosophy contends that this is an illusion. From the Buddhist perspective of "dependent origination" and *karma* (cause and effect) all phenomena arise as the result of the interplay of numerous cause-and-effect relationships. All things in the world are not only interrelated, but also impermanent; and always being in a state of change, they lack "inherent existence." In other words, "Upon examining the ultimate nature of reality, Buddhist philosophers have concluded that things lack inherent existence, that is they do not have self-defining, self-evident characteristics. This is because if we search for the essence of matter in whatever object it may be, we discover that it is unfindable" (Dalai Lama, Benson, Thurman, Gardner, & Goleman, 1991).

In order to demystify this perspective, one might consider the assumptions of string theory in quantum physics, wherein matter, ultimately, can be reduced to energy and movement (Dalai Lama, 2005; Greene, 1999). Similarly, the "Two Truths" working hypothesis can be viewed through the neural network and neuroscientific paradigm, which explains all human phenomenology as arising from spreading activation across a vastly complex network of nodes (LeDoux, 2002). The cognitive scientist and biologist Francisco Varela (2000) has suggested that mindfulness training, and the related affective phenomenon of arising compassion, may represent a form of "neurophenomenology" that allows us to "cut the chain" of conditioned perceptions, revealing a conscious experience of our embodied cognition as an instantiate and self-referential aspect of a vast, perhaps infinite, network of "interbeing." According to Varela, the human mind is an emergent property resulting from the complex organization of embodied cognition, wherein "the organism as a meshwork of entirely co-determining elements makes it so that our minds are literally inseparable, not only from the external environment, but also from our bodies, what Claude Bernard called the *milieu interieur*, the fact that we have not only a brain but an entire body" (Varela, 2000, p. 73).

The broad, interconnected perspective suggested by the theory, neuroscience, and practice of mindfulness and compassion-focused disciplines has far-reaching clinical implications. The clinician employing mindfulness training, compassionate mind training, or interventions aimed at fostering decentering from the content of negative cognitions is actually drawing the patient's awareness toward a more functional, workable experience of themselves as an interactive part of a living process, moment by moment. Practitioners of mindfulness and compassionate mind training disciplines are deploying their attention in a way that may activate a species-preservative network of neural activity that promotes intrapersonal attunement and neural integration. In doing so, they contact a core mode of being, which presents itself as fundamental, liberating, and awe-inspiring. Indeed, the scientific examination of mindfulness may be the beginning of a clinical neurophenomenology of a new model of mental health. Employing mindfulness training as a context for the subsequent cultivation for compassion for the self and others, a radical sanity may begin to be approached that involves a transcendent sense of self and contact with the present moment, both of which have been established as psychological processes that contribute to psychological flexibility and well-being (Hayes et al., 1999). Historical Buddhist philosophical and technical writings point to an inevitable emotional emergent property of this practice, this being the arising of the *bodhicitta*, the altruistic aspiration for the cessation of suffering for all beings. This aspiration can be construed as an abundant compassion emerging from the intellectual and experiential knowledge of the intimate interconnection of all phenomena. Compassion and mindfulness may in this way be viewed as co-creating one another. Our practice of mindfulness creates a meta-awareness and a flexible focused attention that can facilitate the cultivation of compassion and engagement with the world through compassionate courage.

The Expanding Spheres of Awareness

The following practice is a mediation and visualization that experientially links the concept of two truths with a direct experience of our connection to all things. Versions of this practice can be found in Japanese Vajrayana Buddhist practices, central Asian meditation disciplines, and even some forms of esoteric Christian practice. It is an example of a globally emergent practice that reminds us of our essential nature. While this practice is routinely used in Japanese Tendai Vajrayana and other advanced Buddhist practices, this is a meditation that has rarely been used in clinical applications. It can facilitate perspective-taking skills, help us decenter from preconceived beliefs about our narrative self, and remind us of our connectedness to all things. In the author's clinical and educational practice, this meditation has been used with advanced students and clients who have achieved many of their initial treatment goals, in order to continually hone their capacities and to deepen their personal practice.

The visualization is intended to help us to "let go of faulty, destructive conceptualizations of the self or small self state" (S. K. Hayes, 1992, p. 51). In this way, a patient may practice flexible perspective taking, distancing him- or herself from identification with his or her self-story and recognizing his or her connection to an experiential sense of self. As flexible perspective taking is an essential component of psychological flexibility, and highly correlated to well-being (Hayes et al., 2006), such a meditation has potential benefit clinically as well as philosophically. Through this practice we can, perhaps, begin to experience ourselves as an extension of a living, dynamic universe, expanding out from and letting go of a fixed sense of self in time and space (S. K. Hayes, 1992).

Guided Instructions

Find a place that is comfortable, quiet, and that will be relatively free from distractions or interruptions. This is a meditation that is typically done in a seated position. You may choose to sit on a straight-back chair with your legs uncrossed, on a meditation cushion, or even on some pillows. The main aim here is to keep your back in a straight yet relaxed posture. This will allow you to take a deep and full breath into the bottom of the lungs. You might want to imagine your spine as a stack of poker chips, or picture a slender thread gently pulling the top of your head to a dignified position, with the neck relatively free from tension. It is good to keep your feet on the floor when sitting in a chair. If you are on a cushion, allow your knees to rest on the floor. In this way, you will feel more grounded and connected to your support.

Begin by practicing deep, soothing, rhythmic breathing, breathing deeply and evenly. Gently begin to notice the warmth that radiates out from the center of your body. See if you can imagine looking deep inside yourself toward the source of that warmth. Looking inward into your core, into the center of your chest, imagining in your heart the tiniest of points of energy and light as the symbolic source of your body's warmth, vitality, and strength.

Continue to focus on this point of light, this small golden point of energy and light at the center of your heart. Breathing in deeply, allowing the air to replenish your body with oxygen and increasing your attention and awareness. As you inhale deeply, fully, imagine this golden-white point of light growing in size, brightness, and illumination. As you exhale, imagine your body releasing elements that it no longer requires. With each exhalation, let go of excess tension, center yourself, and sustain your focus on the expanded point of light.

Continue to observe this light growing to become a sphere of glowing warm energy in the center of your heart and body. As you breathe, allow this light to continue to radiate and grow. See if you can enjoy the sensation as it warms your heart and then your entire core, and moves up and down to encompass your entire body with golden-white light and mellow, soothing warmth. Perhaps you may want to smile slightly to yourself as you notice the benefits of this light as it restores, energizes, and balances the processes and functioning of your body.

Gently allow this orb of warmth and light to expand from your body, from your skin and outward to form a sphere of energy with you at its center. This golden-white light radiating gently out from your core, from your head and shoulders, and out from under you into the earth beneath your feet. As you continue to focus on the warmth of the glowing sphere around you, allow yourself to imagine this globe as your expanded presence in this space you have chosen to practice. With the inhale, visualize this personal presence reaching out, growing in even more directions, filling up the room with the strength of your vibrancy, warmth, kindness, and stability. As best you can, imagine all things enclosed in your sphere of expanded awareness are enriched, soothed, and unified with your presence and essential nature. Allow yourself to extend this caring, encouraging connectedness to all that lies within this sphere. As if all those "other" things and beings are a part of this expanded single energy with your heart at its center.

On your next inhale, visualize this globe of presence and light grow and move through the walls, outward, beyond the limits of this building, enfolding the whole of the street, the neighborhood, and the local community. Allow yourself to find enjoyment in the expanding care, warmth, and encouragement as it surrounds all beings, animals, plants, events, people, and things that you passed on your way to this place today and perhaps on other days. See if you can feel this expansion and the sensation of an abundance of energy, light, and space for all. Visualize this entire community brighten, heal, and evolve, supported within the influence of your presence and brightness. Allowing yourself to care deeply for everything within this sphere, taking pleasure in all the joys and feeling empathy and care for all misfortune.

Continue to breathe and grow your circle of presence and expanding awareness to include your entire city and state (or geographical region), engulfing and connecting with everything within the care and protection of your radiating consciousness and light. See all of this area of the world as unified in your spacious compassionate presence.

Imagine your globe of consciousness growing to enclose the entire continent, brightening everything above, below, and on your continent. The earth, plants, water, animals, men and women are all connected to and enhanced by this emerging awareness and energy. Imagine all the warmth, courage, energy, love, and strength you would want for yourself, being offered to you and all that your sphere includes. All move in the direction of wellness, peace, and balance.

Expand your presence to encircle and brighten the entire earth. See the whole planet as included in this connected and expanded awareness and intention. Expand your nurturing light to engulf the whole world, its atmosphere, and its moon. Allowing everything in this world to be cared for and to become a part of this intention and energy.

Allow yourself to grow your presence to take in all of the solar system and its forces, objects, and space. Imagine your sphere connecting in an expanding "oneness" all that is within your solar system.

As you inhale, expand to incorporate the Milky Way. Imagine that your awareness and presence has now grown into a sphere of light and warmth big enough to incorporate your entire part of the universe.

Allow yourself to feel the magnitude of this orb of presence and awareness, large enough to enclose this galaxy and the next galaxies in all directions until you have embraced the entire universe. Imagine yourself as being a part of and caring for all that exists in this universe. This sphere of light and warmth is connected to and found within all universal things, past, present, and future. This awareness is the awareness of all space, of all time. This presence is the presence of all that could be. See if you can enjoy this expanded awareness and connectedness. Perhaps, smiling to yourself as you spend a few moments basking in the image of being unified with and deeply caring for "all-that-is," all that is a part of "you."

From this experience and image of being a compassionate protector of all existence in the universe, slowly inhale deeply and begin to reverse the direction of your visualization. Slowly begin to bring in your awareness and presence from the very edges of the universe, beginning to move back in. Gently breathe as you imagine tightening this sphere of awareness, slightly reducing your view of outer space, drawing your awareness toward the center.

As you inhale and exhale, continue bringing your awareness inward, imagining the reducing range of your strong and radiant orb of light and warmth. Focus the sphere in through the galaxy and the solar system. Now finding your presence and light surrounding the edges of the earth's atmosphere. Continuing to breathe and imagine the reducing in circumference to your continent, then state, city, and then your neighborhood, and the building in which you are practicing. Pulling in the reach of your light and consciousness into the walls of the room you have chosen for practice, and to the edges of your personal space. Now allow the sphere to encompass just your body.

Take a moment to enjoy this warmth and radiance surrounding and supporting you and then continue to tighten your awareness further toward the center. See if you can feel the sphere of energy condense within you, smaller and smaller now, only filling your chest and core, and then only your heart.

As much as you can, watch the light of your presence tighten to a pinpoint size and then get so small it seems to "vanish" deep into your very center, the core of your being. Although it may seem undetectable, the potential and capacity of your awareness and outreach is always there to offer a bridge or link between you as an individual and you as a self-aware facet of an infinite, living, and diamond-like universe. How near and how far will you allow your awareness and consciousness to connect and assume responsibility?

After spending a few more moments with this image, begin to let it all go. Breathe slowly and deeply, gently allowing your breath and attention to return to settle on the physical sensations in the abdomen. Now, with the next in-breath, allow your attention to focus on the sounds that surround you in the room. Next, bring the attention to the sounds outside of the room. Following this, allow your attention to gently settle on the sounds even farther away than that. Giving yourself a few moments to gather your attention and orientation to your presence on the mat, you can open your eyes, and resume your daily activities.

Cultivating the Compassionate Mind in Buddhist Psychology and Cognitive-Behavioral Therapy

The Compendium of Perfect Dharma reads, "O Buddha, a Bodhisattva should not train in many practices. If a Bodhisattva properly holds to one Dharma and learns it perfectly, he has all the Buddha's qualities in the palm of his hand.
And, if you ask what that one Dharma is, it is great compassion."
—KAMALASHILA (as quoted in Dalai Lama, 2001, p. 43)

DEEPENING OUR UNDERSTANDING OF COMPASSION

The English word "compassion" represents the combination of two Latin roots: *com*, meaning "together" and *pati*, meaning "to suffer," and it is defined as "sorrow for the suffering of another or others, accompanied by an urge to help" (*Webster's New World Dictionary*, 1988, p. 284). This definition, which is consistent across both Western and Buddhist contexts, has two crucial components, which correspond to the "two psychologies" of compassion.

First, compassion requires sensitivity to suffering. This sensitivity means that when we are experiencing compassion, we have a keenly focused present moment awareness of the presence of suffering in ourselves or others. Second, this sensitivity is accompanied by a motivation to act. Specifically, when we experience compassion, we are motivated to do something to alleviate or prevent the suffering we encounter in the world.

Through our experience of compassion, the pain that we witness pains us. Most obviously, this means that our experience of pain in another will cause us pain, in both an affective and sympathetic sense as well as in an empathic and cognitive understanding of what it would be like to feel the pain that we witness. In a deeper sense, however, our ability to shift our perspective can allow us to view ourselves as we might view another person. At such times, we imagine what it would be like to witness our own suffering from the outside. As such times, we are capable of self-compassion, and we are moved to engage with the suffering we witness within ourselves. Just as in the classic cognitive therapy exercise, known as "The Double Standard" technique, in a time of distress we might ask ourselves, "What would I say to a very good friend who was struggling with this issue? If someone I felt great loving-kindness for was facing this issue, and talking to him- or herself in this way, what would I want to say to help him or her to move through this pain?"

Compassion in Buddhist Psychology

According to Buddhism, compassion is an aspiration, a state of mind, wanting others to be free from suffering. It's not passive—it's not empathy alone—but rather an empathic altruism that actively strives to free others from suffering. Genuine compassion must have both wisdom and loving kindness. That is to say, one must understand the nature of the suffering from which we wish to free others (this is wisdom), and one must experience deep intimacy and empathy with other sentient beings (this is loving kindness).

—DALAI LAMA (2005, p. 49)

If we were to identify a single virtue most central to Buddhist psychology, it would be compassion. It is said that the historical Buddha did not consider compassion to be a part of Buddhist practice, but to be *all* of Buddhist practice (Makransky, 2012). Compassion is described as playing a vital role throughout the entirety of the journey described in biographies of the historical Buddha. Moved by the suffering of those he saw, the Buddha abandoned a life of privilege in favor of the attempt to understand and find freedom from suffering. Compassion propelled him through years of asceticism as he followed different teachers and traditions in his quest. Finally, once the Buddha had found his own answers, compassion compelled him to spend the remainder of his life teaching others.

This story of the Buddha, regardless of its historical veracity, is mythopoetic, archetypal, and of profound global significance in terms of how civilized human beings have come to understand a personal journey to address the very real problem of human suffering in this lifetime. Compassion is at the center of the archetypal journey of the historical Buddha, just as it is at the center of the personal path of each clinician who reads these words. Rather than view compassion as a soft option, or in blurry and vague terms, the mission that falls to us is to comprehend the dynamic, active processes engaged in compassion, as manifested in the consultation room as well as in the daily lives of everyone we know.

At present, Buddhism survives in three major denominations, these being *Theravada*, "The Elder Vehicle," *Mahayana*, "The Great Vehicle," and *Vajrayana*, "The Diamond Vehicle." While the forms of practice may differ in these schools of thought, compassion retains its central role throughout the three. In Buddhist psychology, compassion (*karuna*) is one of the "immeasurable qualities" (*Brahmaviharas* in ancient Sanskrit), which practitioners strive to cultivate in their pursuit of enlightenment. Our current conceptualizations of compassion involve all of the elements of compassion that are described as these "immeasurable" qualities. A therapist practicing Buddhist-informed CBT will be working with all of these human experiences at one time or another. After the desire for others to cease suffering, compassion, or *karuna*, the other immeasurables are loving-kindness, sympathetic joy, and equanimity (Bodhi, 2005; Das, 1997). We can think of loving-kindness as the mirror image of compassion: where compassion is wishing others to be free from suffering, loving-kindness is wishing others to be happy. Sympathetic joy means that we take joy in others' benefit and successes, not simply our own. Finally, equanimity means that we abide in calm clarity and wisdom, and do not favor some beings over others: the experiences of compassion, loving-kindness, and sympathetic joy are applied in relation to all. While there are four different abodes, they all may be viewed as aspects of compassion as it is deployed in Buddhist psychology-informed CBT. As our patients train their minds in compassion, their sensitivity and motivation to address human suffering where they encounter it can grow (*karuna*). Similarly their warm, supportive desire for the well-being and flourishing of self and others (*metta*) is enhanced through practice. Stepping back from overidentification with the contents of consciousness (mindfulness) affords the ability to take deep, empathic pleasure in the well-being of others (*mudita*), and to view our own flourishing with less attachment, as we may view that of another. This coming together of these processes naturally flows into an experience of equanimity (*uppekha*), wherein our fusion with our self-narratives falls away, and our biases toward self-focus become less central. We see our common humanity, and are moved to extend compassion even to those parts of ourselves, and to those others, whom we initially held in contempt.

Generations of Buddhists have asserted that the four aspects of compassion might be the central ingredients of our individual evolution. Looking more closely, we see that loving-kindness is the central focus of the most widely practiced Buddhist meditation on compassion, the *metta* meditation. This practice has guided the cultivation of compassion for millions of Buddhist psychology practitioners for thousands of years. Recently, some CBT practitioners have so valued and widely deployed training in *metta* that the meditative practice has earned its own cognitive-behavioral acronym. Specifically, several CBT practitioners have dubbed the practice the LKM (loving-kindness meditation practice) (Frederickson et al., 2008). In years to come, this LKM will likely retain a central role in the integration of Buddhist psychology and CBT.

The Metta Meditation: The LKM

The following meditation is a Western translation of the classic *Metta* meditation. Many of the practices that are used throughout CBT-based adaptations of compassion training will use variations on the *Metta* meditation theme. A range of current CBT applications have used the Loving-Kindness meditation, and a recent comprehensive literature review has found that the adoption of loving-kindness training as a process can be a useful augmentation to current CBT protocols (Hofman et al., 2011). ACT, CFT, and CBT integrated with the work of Barbara Fredrickson are particularly clear examples of CBT practices working with loving-kindness practices (Hofman, 2012; Tirch, Schoendorf, & Silberstein, 2014). While this meditation is not prescribed for a specific diagnosis, clients who struggle with shame-based difficulties may be particularly good candidates for such a line of work.

In the LKM we are presented with a unique example of a prescientific intervention, designed *specifically* to foster more adaptive emotion regulation and to address anxiety and aggression, that is now being supported by empirical evidence. The practice is very simple, and involves the meditator visualizing him- or herself as innocent, and deserving of compassion and care. When this image is formed, the meditator then begins to recite a phrase that aspires to self-compassion, such as "May I be filled with loving-kindness, may I be peaceful and at ease, may I be well." Accompanying this visualization and recitation, the person engaged in this training also aims to foster a direct sensory experience of compassion and love by focusing on sensations in the body that are related to such emotions. This is practiced regularly for about 30 minutes, over a long period of time, traditionally. After self-compassion is generated, this exercise can be used to cultivate compassion for others, even those toward whom one might have anger or ill-will. In this way, as the patient remains engaged with this meditative practice, as much as he or she can, he or she is gradually habituating to the experience of compassion, and increasing his or her ability to flexibly remain in the presence of the difficult feelings that may arise when he or she directs compassionate attention inward.

The intervention itself follows the basic format of the mindfulness practices that are explained in detail earlier in this text. The therapist will guide the patient through the steps of this exercise, which the patient can later follow either from memory, from having approximately memorized the instructions in a patient handout, or from following a recorded guided "loving-kindness" meditation. There are several examples of guided "loving-kindness" meditations available. It may also be advisable for the therapist to record the guided meditation as it takes place "in session" and to give the patient a copy of this recording. Like mindfulness practices, this meditation should take place in a quiet, safe place, with the patient seated on a meditation cushion or a straight-backed chair, or lying flat on the floor.

Guided Instructions

Loving-kindness is a quality that can help us to abide with difficult experiences, rather than struggle against that which we cannot change. This quality of warm, compassionate regard for the self and others is also associated with the cultivation of a sense of well-being that can translate into positive actions taken in the service of a meaningful and rewarding life. The meditation we are about to embark upon may be viewed as one of the most ancient and enduring "mental health" practices in human history. For over 2,500 years, people have sat silently, and drew their attention to the cultivation of love and appreciation for themselves and all living beings in this way. As you take your seat to begin this meditation, take a moment to realize that you share an aspiration with centuries of fellow travelers, as you embark upon your own private journey toward compassion. Set aside about 20 minutes to engage in this exercise at first; later on you may want to devote a little more time to it, or let it go entirely. Unlike some other meditation exercises, this exercise involves a focus on specific emotions and specific images. At first, this kind of exercise might elicit feelings different from those you are aiming to explore. It may even bring about some frustration. All of this is okay. As best as you can, allow yourself to be kind and patient with yourself. You are exploring ideas and practices that may be very new and different to you. The kindness and patience that you can direct toward yourself in the face of frustration can provide yet another opportunity to practice and deepen your capacity for self-compassion.

As you begin, take a seat on a straight-backed chair or meditation cushion. Just as you would in a mindfulness meditation exercise, bring your attention to the flow of the breath. Make any small adjustments that you might need to make in order to be as comfortable as possible. As the exercise proceeds, if you need to adjust your posture from time to time, that is okay. Bring part of your attention to the flow of your breath. As much as you can, without judgment, just observe the breath as you breathe in and breathe out. Gather your awareness of the physical act of breathing, and simply follow the flow of the breath, moment by moment.

Form an image of yourself in your mind. Imagine that you are seated in the same posture that you now sit in. You may wish to picture yourself as a child. You are innocent, and worthy of love and compassion in this image. If you do not wish to imagine yourself as a child for this exercise, simply imagine yourself as you are now, but held in a kind, loving appreciation. Recognize, just for a moment, that all beings wish to be happy and free from pain. All people have an inborn motivation to feel loved and held in kindness and acceptance. Realize that it is all right for you to wish to be happy and free from suffering. As you do this begin to silently repeat the following phrase, "May I be filled with loving-kindness. May I be well. May I be peaceful and at ease. May I be happy." Hold the image of yourself in your mind as you repeat this. Allow the rhythm of repetition to flow with your breath. Allow yourself to engage in this exercise gently, but with a spirit of immovability. Allow your "heart" to open to the meaning of these words. As you continue through this exercise, let yourself blend the feeling of being loved and held in unconditional kindness with the flow of the words themselves.

Whenever your mind has wandered, which is an inevitable behavior of the mind, gently direct your mind back to the phrase, the image, and the feeling of loving-kindness. "May I be filled with loving-kindness. May I be well. May I be peaceful and at ease. May I be happy." It is natural that distractions will come and go. Practice a warm acceptance of yourself as you proceed through this exercise, and allow yourself to gently return your attention to the repetition as many times as is necessary. When the time that you have allowed for this exercise has past, simply let the phrase go. As you exhale, let the image of yourself and the deliberate focus on feelings of warmth and compassion go as well. Allow yourself to simply be with the flow of your breath. Breathing in, knowing that you are breathing in. Breathing out, knowing that you are breathing out. As you exhale, allow your eyes to open, and let go of this exercise.

Used with permission, from Leahy, Tirch, and Napolitano (2012). Copyright by The Guilford Press. In turn, the exercise was based on many sources on *metta* meditation, including the writings of Kornfield (1993) and Kabat-Zinn (1990).)

MAHAYANA BUDDHISM AND THE *BODHISATTVA* IDEAL

It is generally accepted that about 500 years after the establishment of the first form of Buddhism (*Theravada*), a radical shift in the aims of

Buddhist practice and philosophy took place among large communities of Buddhist practitioners. This shift resulted in a new school of *dharma* practice, which became known as the "Great Vehicle," or *Mahayana*. It is unclear exactly what promoted this shift; however, we do know that instead of *Mahayana* practice beginning as a discrete and separate sect, this second major variation of Buddhist practice began simply as a difference of emphasis and philosophy within the *Theravada*. Many of the roots of *Mahayana* practice developed along the Silk Road in what was known as the Kushan Empire. Art from this region, as well as other elements of culture, involve a blend of Hellenic, Buddhist, Chinese, and other regional influences. This reflects a broadening understanding of the world, and a shift from a predominantly ascetic ideal and method, to an engaged form of Buddhism that is more situated in social behaviors. Similarly, the philosophy of the *Mahayana* involves a shift of emphasis from the pursuit of individual enlightenment for the good of a single person to an ideal that involves awakening our minds so that we might contribute to the cessation of suffering of all beings, in all times.

Mahayana philosophy emphasizes the interconnectedness and unity of all phenomena, and posits that such interdependent origination contributes to a deep motivation to alleviate the suffering we encounter in any all sentient beings. In the *Mahayana* branch of Buddhism, we can consider compassion to be the fuel that carries one down the pathway of enlightenment. In a text called *The Great Treatise on the Stages of the Path to Enlightenment*, the Tibetan sage Tsong-Kha-Pa (founder of the Dalai Lama's school of Tibetan Buddhism, and indeed the first Dalai Lama) famously establishes compassion as the central valued aim in Buddhist psychology. This effectively represents the foundation of compassion as the key psychological process to be trained and cultivated by centuries of practitioners of the *dharma*. Kha Pa quotes Chandrakirti, his predecessor in the *Mayahana* tradition, as follows:

> Compassion alone is regarded as the seed of a Conqueror's excellent harvest,
> As water for its development,
> And as the maturation in a state of long enjoyment.
> Therefore at the beginning I praise compassion.
> —Tsong-Kha-Pa (2002, p. 30)

In emphasizing compassion in this way, the founding and first Dalai Lama is urgently and poetically reminding us that compassion is key to the pursuit of freeing ourselves and others from suffering on all stages of the path. Just as in the case of the biographical myth of the historical Buddha, compassion must be present in the beginning, middle, and end of our efforts as well. In this way, compassion is the seed, the water, and the maturation, all in one. Interestingly, this resonates with the idea that compassion can serve as both a process variable and an outcome variable in psychotherapy research and practice. Compassion has been, understandably, very tricky to assess and measure accurately as a result. Perhaps using the term "immeasurable" to describe compassion may seem prescient to 21st-century psychologists. Similarly, it is taught that in order to progress along the Buddhist path to enlightenment, one must cultivate both wisdom and method, both theory and practice. Thus, the *Mahayana* calls for us to be true scientist-practitioners, and the call is for our work to focus on compassion (Sopa & Newman, 2008).

As the *Mahayana* evolved into a school of its own, the ideal that was pursued by monks and laypersons alike shifted from individual enlightenment to becoming a *Bodhisattva*, or "awakened being." Hence, the term *Bodhisattva* refers to beings who dedicate themselves to freeing not only themselves from suffering, but all other beings with them. *Bodhisattvas* are seen as being the principal heirs of the Buddha (Dalai Lama, 1994), and the living personification of compassion. From the Buddhist perspective (which traditionally included reincarnation), *Bodhisattvas* would do anything possible to free others from suffering, even delaying their own liberation, and instead choosing to be reborn again and again so that they may continue to work on behalf of other beings. Outside of the cultural context of a belief in reincarnation, fundamentally the *Mahayana* encourages all beings to pursue becoming a *Bodhisattva* in this lifetime. Essentially, this simply means devoting one's life to practicing mental training and making a commitment to seek the liberation of suffering for all beings through action. There are specific areas of training (the six perfections) and a specific set of vows (the *Bodhisattva* vows) that accompany committed action on this path. However, the core of the practice goes deeper than the form of the vows or historically situated trainings. *Bodhisattvas* are individuals who use these methods to promote and evoke the aforementioned capacity of mind known as *Bodhichitta*.

For CBT purposes, we can think of *Bodhichitta* as referring to a sincere, overarching motivation to attain freedom from suffering in order to benefit all beings and, in turn, to help free them from suffering. It is a wish that involves the activation of all of the attributes and skills of the compassionate mind, and that can reorganize our minds and our lives toward compassionate action. This is the wish that propels the *Bodhisattva* toward enlightenment, and its root is compassion (Pelden, 2007). According to Buddhist psychology, awakening the compassionate mind fundamentally alters the experience and possibilities of the person on the *Bodhisattva* path.

With the *Mahayana*, we can see how the centrality of empathy and interconnectedness began to shape Buddhist psychology. However, compassion was present at the beginning of Buddhist psychology, as Sidartha Gotama began the lifelong journey that would bring him to an "awakened" state of mind. Furthermore, compassion is present today, as a characteristic that contemporary Buddhist practitioners strive to cultivate above all else, as they pursue their own paths.

Karma and Compassion

If we look at the goals of Buddhist practice, we can see why compassion is so important. One aspect of Buddhism that has made its way into mainstream culture is *karma*, which we can think of as the law of cause and effect. Some may think of *karma* in the manner of a cosmic scorecard that magically keeps track of our actions and ensures that they "come back to us." Nonetheless, this supernaturally romantic idea isn't what is taught in Buddhism. Rather, we can recall from our earlier discussions that the Buddhist view of reality is defined by a constant interplay of causes and conditions in which nothing is "solid" and everything is interdependent. From this perspective, all of our thoughts, emotions, and actions function as causes that ripen over time to impact both the world around us and our own cognitive tendencies. So, our thoughts and actions today don't simply impact our current reality—they create the conditions that will come to define our future reality as well. This is particularly true at the level of the mind, which Buddhists see as the real source of all happiness and suffering. Buddhist teachings long ago forecast what modern neuroscience has confirmed (and which every student who has ever studied for an exam or practiced for a recital or sporting event already knew, at least implicitly)—that thinking and behaving in certain ways today increases the probability of thinking and behaving in similar ways in the future. While Buddhists may explain this in terms of planting seeds that ripen in the mind, and neuroscientists may speak in terms of implicit memory and strengthening neural networks over time, the outcome is the same: the thoughts, emotions, and actions we experience and cultivate today directly and indirectly shape our experience of reality in the future. This is *karma*.

Given the perspective of *karma*, the Buddhist emphasis on cultivating virtuous thoughts, emotions, and actions is more pragmatic than it is lofty; if our current thoughts, emotions, and behaviors act as the causes and conditions that shape our future reality, then it makes sense to cultivate those that will shape a reality that is happy, free of suffering, and prepares us to help ourselves and other beings. This perspective is greatly empowering because it firmly places us as the architects of our own future. In this role, the choices of the present are doubly weighted—if we indulge in petty jealousy in the present, it makes us more likely to experience jealousy and dissatisfaction in the future; if we think, feel, and act kindly in the present, we are more likely to experience kindness later on. These moments matter, as each one of them shapes who we will be, and the extent to which we will suffer, later on (and from the Buddhist perspective of rebirth, what our future lives will look like).

As compassionate understanding, compassionate motivation, and compassionate action are keys to transforming not only the mind, but our cause-and-effect patterns of interacting with the totality around us across time and space, we can see why compassion is so highly revered in Buddhism. At the level of specific behavior, compassion serves to keep the Buddhist practitioner committed and on-task. To the uninitiated, Buddhism can seem to have an overwhelming number of lists of virtues that one needs to cultivate (and, to be fair, Buddhism does involve lots of lists—very likely as mnemonic devices to preserve teachings that relied on oral transmission alone for many hundreds of years). However, we can see compassion as tying them all together. If we are honestly able to cultivate and maintain *Bodhichitta*, or "great compassion," the sincere wish that all beings (including ourselves) be free from suffering, and the will to accomplish that for them—the other activities may naturally fall into place. We will naturally pursue a policy of nonharm because we won't be able to bear the idea of causing suffering. We will naturally pursue wisdom because wisdom is required to free us and other beings from suffering. We will naturally cultivate virtues like generosity, patience, empathic joy, and equanimity, as each of these provides yet another vehicle for actualizing our compassionate intent. Doing all of this is hard work, and it requires a powerful motivation to keep at it when the going gets tough. From the Buddhist perspective, this powerful motivation is compassion.

The role of compassion in freeing us from suffering isn't just as a motivator, however. From the Buddhist perspective, suffering is the product of obsessive tendencies to cling and to crave, and in particular, to cling to ideas of the self—for example, by constantly examining, evaluating, and comparing the self to others. Compassion takes the focus away from the neurotic self, and places it squarely upon the individual or individuals that are being cared for. With compassion, our focus shifts from an obsessive focus on the self that keeps us criticizing and aggrandizing ourselves, competing with and comparing ourselves to others, and instead directs our energy toward recognizing suffering, courageously facing it head on, and doing what is necessary to address it. It shifts us from a perspective of "Am I under attack?", "Am I important enough?", "Do I have enough?", "Am I better than him?", "Am I loved?", to one of "This being (or I) is (am) hurting. What would be helpful in this situation? What would be the most skillful thing to do?"

In the neuroscience-based model of compassion found in CFT, we understand compassion to be a powerful evolved mode of mind that informs the quality of our experience, action, and attention (Gilbert, 2009a). Rather than imagining this as an evolutionary theory that stands in contrast to Buddhist theory, we can view the lens of evolutionary science as clarifying the focus of our understanding of *karmic*, literally translated as "causal," relationships describing the dynamics of our living universe. In this model the common human experience of emotional suffering is seen as being directly related to powerfully evolved emotion-regulation systems, which are at once somewhat ill-suited to the current human social environment and which interact in ways that can both produce tremendous emotional pain and prolong it over time. As noted, emotion regulation is mediated by three evolved emotion systems: one focused on responding to threats, one focused on pursuing and attaining resources, and one that helps us to feel safeness and contentment in the context of affiliative relationships. These systems are involved in powerful emotional responses (e.g., fear, anger, anxiety, ambition, lust, quiescence, calm) that organize our minds in very different ways—involving distinct patterns of thinking, imagery, motivation, emotional experience, and bodily sensation— patterns of organization that can serve to keep us trapped in the emotion we're experiencing if we don't have awareness of the process. In a sense, evolution has blessed and cursed us with very tricky brains, shaped by attachment and social learning histories. This can lead to tremendous suffering when combined with the inevitable difficulties we will face in life. Like Buddhist psychology, 21st-century compassion psychology aims to systematically help patients to understand the dynamics and difficulties created by their human nature (i.e., their evolved brains), and then helps them to develop compassionate capacities for working with difficult emotions, regardless of whether compassion is directed inward or outward.

Visualizing and Manifesting Our Compassionate Self: The CFT Compassionate Self Exercise

For centuries, practitioners of Tibetan Buddhism and Japanese *Vajrayana* Buddhism have deliberately practiced imaging themselves as being an embodiment of an enlightened and compassionate presence. In Japanese, the practice known as *Sanmitsu*, or "three secrets," represents an intentional coordination of "thought, word, and deed" in order to embody and manifest particular qualities of the enlightened mind. Certain tools, which could be considered to be discriminative stimuli, are used to facilitate a deep experience of immersion in the consciousness of a personification of the awakened mind, such as the compassionate mind. For example, in Buddhist art there are paintings known as *mandala*, which display the Buddha and other mythological beings within a series of circles. These mandala represent a map of the inner world of a human being and are symbolic of the various aspects of our personalities: of our wisdom, our rage, our joy, and even our lust. The mandala or other such images can be used as part of a *sanmitsu* meditation that employs visualization, sound (usually a chanted series of syllables known as *mantra*), and physical gestures (often small hand gestures known as *mudra*) to help evoke the various parts of ourselves so that we may come to terms with all aspects of our being, and from a broader perspective. The idea is that if we focus our thoughts (in terms of mental images), words (mental or verbal phrases with special meanings) and deeds, in the form of unique gestures that connect us with a particular experience, we can then later recall certain aspects of our personality that may help us to transcend suffering.

Many forms of CBT have employed imagery to evoke certain experiences. CFT in particular has drawn upon its overt Buddhist psychology influences to make the use of imagery central in the cultivation of compassion (Gilbert, 2009b). Beyond Buddhist psychology, Paul Gilbert has also used extensive consultation with method acting instructors to find culturally consonant ways of accessing certain emotional states and states of being through memory, sense, and attention. Exercises like the Compassionate Self Exercise have been researched and applied in the treatment of a range of psychological problems such as depression and anxiety, shame-based difficulties, psychosis, smoking cessation, eating disorders and other treatment aims (Tirch & Gilbert, 2014). Much like cognitive restructuring or exposure, systematically training the mind in compassion is a process that may have benefits transdiagnostically. Following a treatment plan that proceeds from a Buddhist-informed or compassion-focused case conceptualization, a clinician may choose to integrate a process of compassionate mind training as a treatment component that runs parallel with the other elements of an evidence-based approach.

This next exercise will help you imagine yourself in a different way from what you might be accustomed to, as if you are an actor who is rehearsing a role in a play or a film. The exercise involves the creation of the personification of your compassionate self who you will meet and who will be happy to see you. This practice, known as The Compassionate Self exercise, is a CFT practice derived from Buddhist psychology and method acting. One of us (D. T.) began his Buddhist training practicing *sanmitsu* visualization in the *Tendai dharma* lineage. When this author encountered the Compassionate Self practice training with Paul Gilbert, he noted a resonance with both decades of *Vajrayana* practice, and the accessibility and simplicity of the imagery work designed for secular, 21st-century people.

Although it may take some gradual practice for patients to become fluent in this practice, it is a foundational imagery exercise for all of the authors, for CFT practitioners, and is increasingly being adapted by ACT practitioners as well.

As we begin to prepare to actually engage in this practice, let's take a moment to think about the qualities of our compassionate self by writing down the qualities you would ideally like to have if you were calm, confident, and compassionate. For our purposes, it doesn't matter at all if you believe you actually have these qualities. We are wondering *what it would be like if you were your compassion self? In this moment, imagine what it would be like to really be your most compassionate version of yourself. How wonderful would it be to actually be that compassionate self? What would you be like? Would you be wise? Would you be strong and able to tolerate discomfort? Would you have warm feelings toward others and toward yourself? Would you feel empathy for someone else's suffering? Would you be understanding of others' faults and foibles, nonjudgmental, and forgiving? Would you have courage?*

Ask yourself how you would picture your most compassionate aspect. Perhaps you might imagine yourself older and wiser, or younger and more innocent. This is *your* exercise, and you are free to embellish and design an image of your compassionate self according to your own desire. In Buddhist psychology, specific archetypal imagery may be used to represent specific mythological *Bodhisattvas*. But in compassion-focused CBT, we are free to create imagery that speaks to our own personal mythology and connects with our own heartfelt wishes.

Guided Instructions

To begin, find a place where you will feel safe and may remain uninterrupted for some time. Ideally, this would be a quiet and special place, such as the one you might use for your mindfulness practice. Begin the exercise as you would the Soothing Rhythm Breathing or similar mindfulness meditations. Allow your eyes to close, bring part of your attention to the soles of your feet as they connect with the floor and to your sit bones on the chair. Allow your back to be straight and to feel supported. Next, partly direct your attention to the flow of your breath in and out of your body; allow it to find its own rhythm and pace. Feel yourself breathe in and breathe out. Continue this breathing uninterrupted until you've gathered your attention and feel focused on the present moment.

We are focusing, here and now, on specific qualities of your compassionate self. Remembering the qualities of your compassionate self, and now imagining that you already have those qualities. Beginning with kindness and the desire to be helpful and supportive. Focus on your motivation and desire to be compassionate, and to contribute to helping yourself and others be free from suffering, to be happy and prosper. As you connect with this compassionate motivation, hold your friendly facial expression, and consider your tone of voice—how you would speak in a compassionate way. For these 30 seconds or so, gently imagine that you have great kindness and the desire to be helpful. Notice how you feel when you imagine yourself in this way.

Remembering that your compassionate self is wise, breathe in, and imagine yourself possessing abiding wisdom and clear seeing; breathe out and let go. Your compassionate self represents and personifies wisdom and understands that life is very hard, and that none of us choose to suffer. Emotional pain and fear is our common bond, and you can sense that this compassionate self has learned through experience that suffering is not our fault. After all, we didn't choose to be here, nor did we choose to evolve with such very complicated brains, filled with strong and confusing emotions and motivations. We didn't choose our personal histories or our painful memories. Knowing all of this, your compassionate self truly understands the difficulty of the life you face and is filled with abundant wisdom. For these 30 seconds or so, gently imagine that you have great wisdom. Notice how you feel when you imagine yourself in this way.

For the next few moments, as you are breathing in and out, imagine what the tone of your voice would be if you were this compassionate self. How would you behave? What would the expression on your face be? Allow yourself to take pleasure in your capacity to share kindness with and care for those around you and yourself. If your mind wanders, as it so often does for all of us, use your next natural inhale to gently bring your attention back to this image of your compassionate self. Breathe into the felt sense of your ability to be compassionate toward yourself, and toward others. Imagine yourself as a completely nonjudgmental person who doesn't condemn, no matter what. Allow yourself to bring to mind the sensory details that you would notice as your compassionate self. What are you wearing? Is your body relaxed and receptive? With body language that signals openness and kindness? Are you smiling? If not, smile now, and at the same time imagine the warmth you feel when you carefully hold an infant. As you breathe in, bring attention into your body, imagine yourself expanding, and welcome your ability to be wise, warm, and resilient.

In this moment, remember that our compassionate self has a deep reservoir of inner strength and the ability to tolerate and contain suffering and distress without being overwhelmed and with immovable compassion and calm, even in the presence of great pain and fear. Your compassionate self is strong, and in this moment, you are strong. For these 30 seconds or so, gently imagine that you have deep and sustaining inner strength. Notice how you feel when you imagine yourself in this way.

Your compassionate self embodies a deep commitment to alleviate your suffering and pain and takes pleasure and satisfaction when you experience joy and happiness. The greatest desire of your compassionate self is to help calm your suffering and anxiety, and to bring you peace, warmth, and contentment.

Imagine that you have a sense of confidence and authority. Feel this dignified, centered authority in your upright body posture. Imagine being able to face suffering and life difficulties with the calm understanding that "whatever is happening, I can work with this too." Keeping your compassionate facial expression and warm tone of voice, think about how you would speak in a compassionate way, how you would move about in the world, expressing your calm confidence and maturity. For the next 30 seconds, gently imagine yourself as this confident, calm, strong, and compassionate authority. Notice how you feel when you imagine yourself in this way.

To develop this practice, imagine that you are looking at yourself from the outside. See your facial expressions, the way you move in the world. Hear yourself speaking to others, noting your compassionate tone of voice. See others relating to you as a compassionate person. See yourself relating to other people in this ideal compassionate way that you are developing. For the next 30 seconds or so, playfully and gently enjoy watching yourself being a compassionate person in the world, and other people relating to you as such.

When ready, return your attention to the present moment, bringing your compassionate presence into the world. As you develop your practice, you can imagine yourself having all those qualities you have been practicing. The more you practice slowing down and imagining being this kind of person in the world, the more easily you may find that you can access these qualities in yourself—and the more easily they will be able to express themselves through you.

Based on practices from Gilbert (2009a), Tirch (2012), and Kolts (2012).

COMPASSION AND ATTENTION

Compassion impacts where our attention is placed, and shapes where it will tend to be drawn in the future: instead of being constantly vigilant to cues and clues about our own social standing (and to things that may threaten it), we are vigilant regarding signs of suffering, and to steps we could take to help alleviate it. It helps us to shift our attention out of the intense but narrow emotions of the moment, reorienting ourselves toward the broader pursuit of freedom from suffering—in the Buddhist view, working to develop an understanding of the ultimate nature of reality. For modern psychologists, this could mean mindfully observing and stepping outside of the mental "crisis of the moment" to consider the situation in relation to one's larger pursuit of a happy, healthy life. The historical Buddha knew what the White Bear Suppression Test and

research on experiential avoidance would confirm better than two millennia later: that if you want to change someone's thinking tendencies, it
doesn't work to tell them to simply stop thinking about the self: attempts
at thought suppression will only increase the frequency of the thoughts
arising (Wegner, Schneider, Carter, & White, 1987). While thoughts are
notoriously resistant to being suppressed, attention is open and available
to be directed and focused, with practice. For the purposes of liberation
from the restrictive grip of mental suffering, what better focus might we
find than self-compassion?

We can see how this works when we contrast the experience of
self-compassion with experiential avoidance, a human tendency that
is linked with a variety of psychological difficulties (Hayes et al.,
1996). With experiential avoidance, one observes emotional pain (or
the potential for it) and recoils, perhaps engaging in a variety of strategies designed to help one escape from or avoid the aversive emotional
experience, some of which are unhelpful and may produce very negative unintended consequences. In contrast, when faced with suffering,
the self-compassionate person can mindfully observe their discomfort
from a kind perspective that sees it in the context of the larger common
human experience, with even their painful emotions being understood
as products of emotion regulation systems that were millions of years
in the making. Rather than being trapped in patterns of thinking and
behavior designed to minimize any contact with the painful emotions,
this individual can accept them, learn that they are capable of experiencing and enduring them, and work to address the factors that serve to
cause or maintain the suffering. Indeed, self-compassion has been found
to be negatively correlated with experiential avoidance. In a study that
followed the self-report of 40 undergraduates over a 1-month period,
Neff and colleagues (2007a) found that an increase in self-compassion
was negatively correlated with thought-suppression strategies. Similarly,
Neff and colleagues (2005) found that self-compassion was negatively
correlated with reported avoidance-based coping strategies in a sample
of 110 undergraduates who had just failed a test. These findings correspond with Neff's early findings (2003a) that self-compassion was negatively correlated with thought suppression and avoidance in a sample of
232 undergraduates.

Our aim in cultivating compassionate attention is not to suppress
a certain set of experiences or to avoid negativity, but to awaken and
activate human capacities that have been designed by evolution to help

us best adapt to and address challenging circumstances. By cultivating compassion and developing what we in the 21st century might call a "mentality of caring" (Gilbert, 2009a), we shift our current attention (and, over time, begin to shape our habitual patterns of future attention) in ways that will naturally tend to reduce the self-focused craving and clinging that Buddhists see as the principle cause of our suffering.

A metaphor used in CFT describes the dynamics of this mental shift by contrasting the impact of teachers that are either critical and irritable or gentle, warm, and compassionate: faced with the first teacher, the student feels "stress, competitive mentality, and rank-focused feelings of being inferior," while the second teacher facilitates feelings of safety, calm, and an enhanced capacity to build and develop positive strategies (Gilbert, 2009a, p. 213). The harsh teacher (or internal self-critic), by causing us to feel threatened, keeps our focus squarely on our fragile self-image; the warm, compassionate teacher helps us to feel safe and allows us to direct our energy to positive thoughts and actions. We can see how the emotional tone of our own internal "teacher" can shape very different mental states in our minds—states that can either encourage us in the pursuit of positive life change, or keep us caught in a shameful self-focus that leads us to feel threatened, helpless, or hopeless. In this example we see another reason why cultivating compassion is important in the Buddhist pursuit of enlightenment; it not only helps us to shift out of the perspective of selfish clinging that can lead to our own suffering, but it leads us to interact with others in ways that help them to do so as well. Finally, it also demonstrates that compassion isn't just about being nice—the encouraging teacher still seeks to motivate his or her students to work hard (even when they're feeling lazy), because the teacher knows that doing so will benefit them.

Like practitioners of the *Bodhisattva* path, cognitive-behavioral therapists are motivated by the compassionate recognition of suffering and the desire to alleviate it. However, in the history of psychological interventions, it could be argued that compassion has served a significant but rather exclusive role as a silent but powerful motivation—felt by the clinician, but rarely spoken of or purposefully cultivated, particularly in terms of formally helping our patients cultivate it in themselves (e.g., in contrast to the way that Buddhist teachers work with their own students). In the world of CBT, however, this is changing.

Behavioral *Bodhisattvas*
Systematic Compassion Interventions

May the frightened cease to be afraid,
And those bound be freed.
May the powerless find power,
And may people think of benefiting each other.
For as long as space endures,
And as long as sentient beings remain,
Until then, may I too abide
To dispel the misery of the world.

— SHANTIDEVA

It might be said that compassion has always been a part of the practice of psychotherapy, else why would one choose to work with patients in the first place? More recently, however, compassion has entered the therapy room in a more formal way—in the form of intervention strategies that seek to help patients develop the capacities for experiencing and directing compassion toward both themselves and others.

CULTIVATING SELF-COMPASSION

In 1989, at one of the first international Buddhist teacher meetings, we Western teachers brought up the enormous problem of unworthiness and self-criticism, shame and self-hatred, and how frequently they arose in Western students' practice. His Holiness the Dalai Lama and other Asian teachers were shocked. They could not quite comprehend the word "self-hatred." It took the Dalai

Lama ten minutes of conferring with Geshe Thubten Jinpa, his translator, even to understand it. Then he turned and asked how many of us experienced this problem in ourselves and in our students. He saw us all nod affirmatively. He seemed genuinely surprised. "But that's a mistake," he said, "Every being is precious!"

—JACK KORNFIELD (2008, p. 27)

Upon reading this quote, one of us (D. T.) couldn't help but reflect that the Dalai Lama and many of his fellow lamas, do, in fact, occupy a position of great esteem and privilege within their social structure. Perhaps, then, their lack of familiarity with self-hostility might be as connected to the social learning histories they have had as it is to their altruistic aspiration for the well-being of all sentient creatures. Nonetheless, our Western social tradition, with its strong emphasis on competition and individual achievement, likely does activate a qualitatively different form of self-aggression than some cultures might. We can find evidence of this in the vast literary, scientific, and dramatic traditions of Western culture, where our heroes often have to face themselves, witness the ways that their hubris has led them to ruin, and then fall into remorse of conscience over the poverty of their nature. Even the doctrine of original sin, so foundational to the Christian tradition, suggests that we are born fallen, and that the blame for our fallen state falls upon us. As we have examined, shame and self-criticism are transdiagnostic processes that are highly correlated with psychological distress (Zuroff, Santor, & Mongrain, 2004), and that can serve as significant obstacles to progress in psychotherapy (Rector et al., 2000). It is no wonder, then, that holding oneself in active kindness in response to persistent self-blame and shame has suggested itself as an avenue for exploration in psychotherapy. Nonetheless, for many of us, the concept of having compassion for one's own self may seem contradictory to what we've learned or thought about compassion in the past. Self-compassion is a new concept for Western psychology, and targeting the development of self-compassion as a key process in psychotherapy is at the frontier of evidence-based practice. However, many prominent Buddhist teachers, such as Pema Chodron (2003) and Thich Nhat Hanh (1973), have emphasized the centrality of self-compassion in the *dharma*. Indeed, self-compassion is conceptually at home within a Buddhist cosmology, where the sense of self is ultimately an illusion. Christopher Germer (2009) has suggested that our society needs an inversion of the Golden Rule, where we begin to treat ourselves the way we would treat a loved one who means the world to us.

Nevertheless, self-compassion remains hard to understand for many. Perhaps this is because in both the East and the West, compassion has primarily been defined and communicated as a state of being moved by the suffering of others and motivated to help them. It's fair to say that the concept of compassion itself initially evolved as an other-directed experience.

Global teachings on compassion, which emphasize focusing on the suffering of others rather than self-focus, may seem to stand in contrast to some Western psychological perspectives that have emphasized the importance of enhancing the self by building self-esteem (Neff, 2003b). In some ways, much of psychology since the mid-20th century has been focused on building the individualistic ego and enhancing how we "esteem" ourselves (Ellis, 2006). This focus stands in contrast to the aims of the Eightfold Path and Buddhist psychology, which would suggest that persons come to liberate themselves from the excessive influence that their self-stories may have over their experience of being. However, there are good reasons to believe that the pursuit of self-esteem may not be the best way to build healthy minds, behaviors, and lives. Recent reviews of the self-esteem literature reveal that there are numerous not-so-positive characteristics associated with the pursuit of high self-esteem, things like the dismissal of negative feedback, taking less responsibility for one's harmful actions, engaging in downward social comparisons that can facilitate prejudice and discrimination, and becoming angry and aggressive toward others who may threaten one's ego (Neff, 2011; Neff & Vonk, 2009). Additionally, in comparison to self-esteem, self-compassion was observed to be more highly related to self-worth, and was less contingent upon the occurrence of particular outcomes (Neff & Vonk, 2009). These findings seem to make a point that is very consistent with Buddhist psychology: building the ego through the development of competitive self-esteem is not the best way to come to peace with oneself or with the world around oneself.

However, when we look at the relatively recent self-compassion movement in psychology, we see that its emphasis is not about deifying the self or competing with others, but learning to extend to oneself the very qualities of compassion that Buddhism seeks to foster in relation to all beings (Neff, 2011). As described earlier, the three elements of self-compassion conceptualized by Neff (2003a) include mindfulness, a sense of common humanity, and self-kindness. Neff has suggested that she directly operationalized self-compassion in this way after studying the writings of Western Buddhist writers on loving-kindness and self-acceptance. Accordingly, the psychology of self-compassion emphasizes the idea that if we are to cultivate compassion for all beings, the self should be included.

Still, one might ask, Why do Western psychologists seeking to apply Buddhist compassion practices with their patients consider focusing on self-compassion in addition to other-directed compassion? Wouldn't doing so merely strengthen the very ego clinging that the Buddha was seeking to help his students overcome? As we will see, the action of the compassionate mind involves the activation of very different emotional, cognitive, and behavioral systems than those involved with social comparison, shame, and threat-based emotions. When we are moved by self-compassion, we are fundamentally shifting away from shame-driven behaviors. Indeed, if we consider some of the dynamics and data regarding the sorts of emotional disturbances that psychology professionals are likely to face, we see that self-compassion makes a good deal of sense. Research reveals that self-criticism, shame, and self-hatred are implicated in numerous emotional and behavioral disturbances, such as depression, anxiety, and self-harm behaviors across diagnostic groups (Gilbert et al., 2010). As the Jack Kornfield quote beginning this section demonstrates, while self-loathing and shame may not have been as much of an issue for the historical Buddha (or possibly for Tibetan monks) due to cultural differences in how one relates to the self, shame and self-loathing play a large role in the Western experience of emotional suffering.

Paul Gilbert spent many years as a shame researcher, and his research demonstrates that shame serves to keep our attention persistently and narrowly focused on the self, both in terms of ongoing internalized negative self-evaluations and in the framing of one's relationships with others in terms of rank-based social evaluations of the self. This social threat-based orientation is distinguished by fears that others are making negative evaluations of us (Gilbert, 1998b). Because social support and human community are so fundamental to our survival, such a narrow, self-focused, threat-based experience of shame is clearly related to narrowing behavioral repertoires and the dominance of destructive emotions. We all desperately fear being completely alone, unprotected and unloved, on some fundamentally human, perhaps nonconscious, level. This experience drives much of our suffering. While it may seem counterintuitive, helping individuals to develop self-compassion may help them to reduce their tendency toward obsessive self-clinging by assisting them in overcoming the shame, ruminative self-criticism, and self-hatred that keeps them trapped in an endless cycle of self-evaluation. In developing compassion toward our own self-experience, we may just be able to free ourselves to move beyond it.

Like compassion that is experienced toward others, self-compassion involves *kindness directed toward the self*. From this kind perspective, we gently open to our own experiences of pain, suffering, or difficulty and allow ourselves to be moved by them, rather than denying pain, pushing it away, or criticizing ourselves for suffering. This kind sensitivity to one's own suffering can flow into taking action to help alleviate the suffering we encounter within ourselves. With self-compassion, we approach our own suffering with gentleness, patience, and a willingness to do what is needed to help (Neff, 2003b).

We have worked with numerous patients who reported having a relatively easy time directing compassion toward others, but a great deal of difficulty bringing the same kind-heartedness to themselves. Where they see the suffering of another as indicative that the person is hurting and could use help, all too often they seem to respond to their own suffering with self-condemnation and shame. The second aspect of Neff's (2003a, 2003b) conceptualization, *common humanity*, helps to address this issue. Rather than viewing one's own suffering as uniquely due to a personal weakness or character flaw, the common humanity aspect of self-compassion involves seeing one's own experiences in the context of the larger body of human experience. Reflecting the teachings of Buddhism, this principle of common humanity involves the direct acknowledgment that if one is to have a human life, one will experience emotional pain, failure, suffering, inadequacies, loss, and a host of other difficulties. This is the common human experience, the price of admission if one is to have human life. In seeing the unavoidable pain involved in this common human experience, one can recognize that having a human life is inherently difficult in many ways, and that all of us, including ourselves, deserve compassion (Neff, 2003b).

With self-compassion, we can recognize our own suffering as a manifestation of our own shared humanity, allowing us to soften our response to it. From a cognitive-behavioral perspective, a Beckian cognitive therapist might see Neff's self-compassion model as involving a form of cognitive restructuring in which negative automatic thoughts that are self-critical and involve core beliefs of isolation and separateness are reframed into thoughts involving self-acceptance and a recognition of suffering as a common human experience. This cognitive shift has the potential to be very powerful, at once assisting the patient in easing up on the critical self-evaluations that may drive much of his or her negative affect, as well as helping him or her to replace a sense of isolation with one of connectedness in which the suffering itself becomes a symbol of the individual's intimate kinship with all other human beings. Over time, a Beckian therapist might expect a gentle shift in the beliefs underlying the patient's difficulties, from "There is something inherently wrong with me, and everything I touch gets messed up" to "Life is difficult for everyone, including me. This is why we need compassion. How can I best take care of myself in this moment?" In considering this situation, we can again see how developing self-compassion can potentially help to weaken the tendency to obsessively focus on the self.

While a Beckian cognitive therapist might seek direct cognitive change from self-critical thoughts to self-compassionate thoughts, third-wave CBT practitioners, such as ACT therapists, might instead seek to help the patient to create conditions in his or her life that fundamentally change his or her relationship with his or her self-criticism. Emphasizing function over form, and targeting contextual variables rather than belief structures, a third-wave CBT therapist might help a patient to cultivate mindful awareness, and to become unstuck from the habitual influence that patterns of thinking might have over his or her behaviors.

Accordingly, the first component of Neff's concept of self-compassion is *mindfulness* itself. As we have discussed, the open, nonjudgmental awareness of mindfulness creates a context in which self-compassion is possible because it allows one to nonjudgmentally observe one's own pain and suffering without identifying with it. In this way, suffering changes so that it is seen as an experience, rather than as a fundamental (flawed, shameful) quality of the self.

At its core, mindfulness involves a quality of open, investigative, nonjudgmental awareness. As such, we can consider that mindfulness itself is perhaps not necessarily either kind or unkind (rather, it is a quality of awareness), but we can see how it supports (and is likely necessary for) the other aspects of self-compassion. As Germer (2009) teaches, however, mindful awareness can be imbued with the quality of warmth, and be used as a vehicle for extending compassion to all experiences encompassed by the awareness. Mindfulness involves opening to one's experience, and seeing it just as it is. Opening ourselves to our own experience is never so difficult as when the quality of that experience is painful, and yet that is just what self-compassion requires and makes possible—a willingness to kindly turn toward the pain. Once we do this, the accepting, nonjudgmental perspective of mindfulness allows one to step out of critical self-evaluation and to recognize the painful experience though the eyes of common humanity—as an experience which is an inherent part of human life, and which can be worked with in a kind, gentle, and patient way. At this point, instead of elaborating on a habitual lifestyle based in avoiding discomfort, we can work with it, kindly, warmly, and courageously. In the words of Christopher Germer (personal communication, April 2013),

> A key element of self-compassion is the shift from mindfulness of experience to mindfulness of the experiencer. When the observer is engulfed in suffering, the observer needs some loving awareness. When the "suffering self" is soothed and comforted, our field of perception naturally reopens to the world around us. In other words, compassion is self-to-self or self-to-other—it's interpersonal, related; it's about connection.

So, we can again note that the way we deploy our attention is a key aspect for the cultivation of compassion.

Soften, Soothe, and Allow

The soften, soothe, and allow exercise is one of several elements of the MSC program that trains patients to directly generate and experience self-compassion. We have chosen this practice as an example because it demonstrates how both mindfulness and self-compassion are dealt with quite directly, warmly, and gently in the MSC program. This exercise can be useful as a daily practice, and can also be deployed as a helpful coping method once a patient has developed familiarity with the processes and experiences it involves. This brief meditation can help us see how we can use mindfulness to make space for our suffering, and how we might apply compassionate attention to our own experience of distress.

Guided Instructions

We begin our practice of gently allowing our experiences by taking a grounded position, with a supple posture and a straight back. Rest upon your chair and allow your breathing to find a natural slow pace and rhythm. When you are ready to begin, take three more breaths in this way, feeling the release of tension with each exhalation.

With the next natural inhale, direct part of your attention to the sensations that are present in the body. Whatever you notice, allow yourself to continue to focus also on the breath, feeling the movement of the belly, and bring open, nonjudgmental attention to the presence of the breath in the area of your heart.

With each inhale, bring compassionate attention into the body, and with each exhale let go of tension, and pay attention to any experience of emotions in the body. What physical sensations, in this moment, feel related to your emotions? Perhaps you have experienced anxiety or distress; if so, this is the time to allow yourself to feel where this emotional experience presents itself as a physical sensation. You may feel anxiety as tension in the chest or throat, for example. Wherever it is, notice it, and bring compassionate attention to this place with each inhale, and feel yourself softening into that space in the body. Imagine this to be similar to applying warmth to stiff or sore muscles. Let go of physically forcing anything at all and repeat the word "soften" over and over again, with the soothing rhythm of the breath. We aren't aiming to suppress or avoid any experience at all here; we are simply bringing mindful and compassionate attention to our emotional and physical experience in this very moment. Stay with this process of softening for a few minutes.

Having softened into this experience, now, if you would like, bring one of your hands to your chest, just over your heart. Feel the warmth of your hand, and through it feel direct kindness and soothing thoughts to yourself. Recognize your struggle, and direct warmth and self-acceptance toward yourself and your experience. Speak kindly to yourself, out loud or in your thoughts, validate your struggle with anxiety and distress, and connect with your compassionate inner voice. You may say something like, "I can see how hard this has been for me now. This pain and these difficult experiences are a part of life. May I grow into greater well-being, peacefulness, and happiness, moment by moment."

Next, gently repeat the word "soothe" in your mind, with part of your attention resting in the soothing rhythm of the breath. You may also choose to imagine the experience of soothing and kindness arriving at that place in the body where you have felt your emotion physically affect you. Notice your inhale and exhale and, as much as you can, remain with this process of soothing for a few more minutes.

As a final step, consciously let go of the need or urge to get rid of your emotional experience. As you exhale, let go of any effort to avoid or suppress your emotion. Having softened into the experience, and brought soothing attention to your struggle, ask yourself to allow your discomfort to be just as it is in this moment. The feeling doesn't need to be pushed away. You are in a safe place, and you can just allow this emotion to be where it is, and for it to come and go in its own time. This time, silently repeat the word "allow" in time with the soothing rhythm of your breath. Just as we have with each gentle step of this practice, stay with this for a few minutes, or however long it feels right to you.

You may choose to silently repeat the words " 'soften, soothe, allow" in your mind as your follow the breath during the last minutes of the exercise. Stay with the breath for as long as you need, resting in the soothing rhythm, and directing mindful, compassionate attention to your emotion.

When you are ready, take one last inhale and then exhale slowly and let go of this exercise altogether, giving yourself credit for having deeply engaged with this practice.

Like our earlier mindfulness exercises, Soften, Soothe, and Allow can be used daily for a period of several days, weeks, or months. This practice, however, may also be used in an abbreviated form to bring compassionate attention into contact with anxiety in the moment it appears to you, wherever you are. This will represent an important transition point, where your practice of mindful awareness begins to move from the meditation cushion to your day-to-day emotion regulation responses. Our next exercises will take this application of mindfulness skills further into the flow of our everyday life.

Based on a meditation found in Germer (2009) and a version of this practice found in Tirch (2012). Used with permission from Little, Brown Book Group.

PRACTICING COMPASSION AS A COMPONENT OF CBT

The fundamental assumption that practicing compassion, mindfulness, and acceptance can help transform the mind and alleviate our suffering unites Buddhist psychology and the current psychological science of self-compassion. Furthermore, such a perspective creates numerous possibilities for enhancing cognitive-behavioral change, and works against our tendency to pursue experiential avoidance. These simple CBT examples share a common intention and rationale with the fundamental assumptions of mindfulness, acceptance, and compassion:

- A therapist encouraging patients to mindfully relax their grip on self-critical thoughts in the presence of social anxiety, through practice.

- A therapist and patient considering, with gentle curiosity, what a range of more self-compassionate and approach-oriented alternatives might be to his or her anxious feelings.

- In session, the therapist and patient practicing mindfulness of difficult emotions, and acceptance of discomfort, as a part of life.

- Pursuing habituation through voluntary exposure to the emotions and the situations that prompt them, seeking a broadening, adaptive series of coping strategies and new behaviors.

In contrast, less self-compassionate and more emotionally avoidant individuals may be reluctant to participate in any strategy that brings them face-to-face with their pain. They may instead engage in a wide variety of less adaptive responses. These may include:

- Denying their suffering altogether.
- Acknowledging their distress for a moment, but quickly shifting to habitual patterns of distraction- and avoidance-based safety behaviors.
- Attributing the fact that they are suffering to undesirable personal characteristics on their own part, and shaming themselves for that "fact."
- Living smaller lives that follow in the behavioral constriction and lost opportunities that habitual experiential avoidance entails.

Considering all of this, an integrative CBT therapist might note how patterns of excessive avoidance and self-criticism might involve the reinforcement of maladaptive self-schemas and thinking patterns. Moreover, an absence of self-compassion might also potentiate failure to habituate to both the challenging emotional state and the stimuli that prompted it. Less self-compassionate people may find themselves stuck in the perpetuation and negative reinforcement of avoidance as a coping strategy. Therefore, the initiation and rehearsal of maladaptive secondary emotional responses directed toward the self (such as self-blame and self-criticism) may be even more painful and enduring than those originally experienced. The behavioral expression of lack of self-compassion or a fear of compassion may also involve noncompliance with therapeutic CBT homework and self-practice. From the perspective of compassion psychology (Gilbert, 2009a), we can see how a self-compassionate perspective can help patients to feel safe in approaching and dealing with life difficulties, where the avoidant alternative can serve to maintain a state of defensive, threat-driven activation that actively works against our therapeutic efforts.

As we have illustrated, the potential benefits of cultivating compassion to transform the mind are not speculations or articles of faith, as there is also a growing body of empirical data that reveal the significant benefits of self-compassion (Neff, 2012). To summarize some of our earlier observations, the literature to date has found that self-compassion, as measured by the Self Compassion Scale (SCS; Neff, 2003a), is associated with lower levels of depression and anxiety, even when controlling for self-criticism and negative affect (Neff, 2003a; Neff, Kirkpatrick, & Rude, 2007). Self-compassion is linked with more adaptive emotional coping, with studies showing that people higher in self-compassion experience greater clarity regarding their feelings and a better ability to repair negative emotional states (Neely, Schallert, Mohammed, Roberts, & Chen, 2009; Neff, Hseih, & Dejithirat, 2005), and engage in a lower frequency of thought suppression and rumination (Neff, 2003a), the latter being a strategy that has long been associated with shame (Cheung, Gilbert, & Irons, 2004; Gilbert, 2003; Tangney, 1995). Finally, self-compassion is associated with a variety of positive states, including feelings of social connectedness, life satisfaction, autonomy, competence, and relatedness (Neff, 2003a; Neff, Pisitsungkagarn, & Hseih, 2008), happiness, optimism, curiosity, and positive affect (Neff, Kirkpatrick, & Rude, 2007).

While several forms of CBT, notably ACT (Forsyth & Eifert, 2007) and DBT (Barley et al., 1993), include modules and techniques that emphasize compassion, an overt focus on compassion as a central change process is mostly lacking across third-wave CBT. Recently, a systematic integration of CFT and ACT has been developed and disseminated (Tirch et al., 2014); however, this unified compassion protocol is still undergoing outcome research. Explicitly bringing compassion training to the forefront of treatment is most evident in the form of two popular treatment models. The MSC program (Neff & Germer, 2011) and CFT (Gilbert, 2009a) are the most overtly compassion-focused therapy modalities that are currently being practiced in affiliation with the broader CBT community. These approaches have several common features, but are also quite different from one another.

Both of these approaches emphasize the purposeful cultivation of compassion, but unlike Buddhism they do not predominantly emphasize compassion in relation to others. Rather, both MSC and CFT emphasize the importance of developing compassion for the self as well. This compassion is not viewed as an emotion in these modalities, but is considered to be an evolved human capacity that organizes the brain and behavior across levels of functioning. By practicing self-compassion, patients train their minds to turn this evolved capacity for compassion toward themselves in order to better address their own emotional suffering and to live lives of greater meaning.

MSC TRAINING

Following on the significant body of empirical work researching self-compassion and having both written self-help books designed to help facilitate self-compassion in individuals who struggle with self-criticism (Germer, 2009; Neff, 2011b), Christopher Germer and Kristin Neff developed the MSC skills training program (Neff & Germer, 2011). The MSC program is strongly influenced by Buddhist psychology approaches, and bears a resemblance to the structure of the MBSR program designed by Jon Kabat-Zinn (1990). This didactic training course specifically teaches participants a number of compassionate mind-training practices derived from those practiced in Buddhist psychology for centuries. The group program runs for eight sessions at 2 to 2½ hours per session, with an accompanying 4-hour retreat. The sessions focus upon the progressive development of skills for fostering compassion toward oneself, with a particular emphasis on developing the qualities of warmth, noncondemnation, and mindful awareness.

The sessions of the MSC program (Neff & Germer, 2011) involve participants in learning various mindfulness exercises, as well as loving-kindness practices that are designed to help develop a sense of affection for themselves and others, extending wishes of kindness, peace, and comfort. As mentioned previously, loving-kindness can be considered the "other side of the coin" in relation to compassion; where compassion involves the wish that oneself and others be free from suffering, loving-kindness involves wishing us and them happiness. We can think of compassion as what happens when loving-kindness meets suffering, and remains loving (Germer, 2009). The MSC program begins by helping participants develop a general understanding of mindful self-compassion and then spends the first three sessions guiding participants through the development of the basic capacities of mindfulness and self-compassion.

The MSC program is intensely skills-based throughout, making extensive use of both in-session exercises (introducing and utilizing numerous exercises, meditations, and informal practices) and daily practices to be done at home. Session 1 focuses on introducing the concept of self-compassion and then guides participants through a number of exercises for cultivating it, such as a "soothing touch" exercise and the Self-Compassion Break, which is included below. Sessions 2 and 3 follow a similar format, using a variety of exercises to assist the participant in the development of mindfulness (with an emphasis on warmth) and loving-kindness. The sessions also involve the exploration of potential obstacles such as experiencing resistance to the exercises and what Germer calls "backdraft" (Germer & Neff, 2011), named for the surge of flame that occurs when a firefighter opens a door (causing oxygen to rush in and feed the fire); this is the tendency for intense and distressing memories and related emotions to emerge when a patient begins to feel heard, supported, safe, and cared for in therapy.

Once the core components of the MSC program have been introduced, Sessions 4 and 5 focus upon applying self-compassion in the context of the patients' daily lives, both pragmatically (Session 4: Finding Your Compassionate Voice) and in terms of helping patients deepen their practice by connecting with their core values and making a commitment to work on them (Session 5: Living Deeply). The 4-hour Retreat Day comes after the fourth or fifth session, and is an opportunity for participants to get a taste of deeper practice, as well as to learn additional meditations such as savoring food, the compassionate body scan, and restorative yoga. The remaining sessions are designed to extend the patients' practice of mindful self-compassion to specific domains with which they may struggle: managing difficult emotions (Session 6) and working with challenges in relationships (Session 7). In addition to applying compassion and mindful acceptance to these issues, specific exercises are introduced for working with particular challenges. For example, Session 6 includes practices for softening toward and working with shame and negative core beliefs, and Session 7 includes practices to help patients understand the emotional dynamics behind having "hard feelings" in relationships, and exercises for forgiving and gradually directing loving-kindness toward challenging others. These practices are based on opening to one's own pain first, with tender, loving recognition. A key aspect of the MSC program is finding a balance between working with difficulties and developing positive strategies that are designed to promote pleasure and happiness. The importance of cultivating strengths and personal resources is reemphasized in Session 8, which focuses on cultivating positive emotions, savoring, and gratitude. An example of such an exercise is the Pleasure Walk, provided in this chapter.

Supporting Evidence for the MSC Program

Initial outcome data provides some support for the effectiveness of the MSC program. In a controlled trial comparing 25 individuals who completed the MSC program with 27 wait-list controls, participants in the MSC group showed significantly greater improvements in self-compassion, mindfulness, compassion for others, and life satisfaction. Additionally, participants in the MSC group showed significant improvements in symptoms of depression, anxiety, stress, and trauma impact relative to controls (Neff & Germer, 2011). Regression data showed that changes in self-compassion predicted significant variance in the changes seen in all of the other variables, and most notably was associated with 48% of the variance in happiness score increases, and 68% of the variance observed in anxiety decreases. These data show that self-compassion interventions, and in particular the MCS training program, have the potential to help us assist psychotherapy patients with some of their most common presenting problems. While this initial trial did involve a nonclinical sample, many of whom had prior experience with meditation, these initial results do support the potential clinical utility of the MSC program specifically, and training in self-compassion more generally. Importantly, these data indicate that interventions that systematically assist patients in developing mindfulness and self-compassion not only help to decrease symptoms of psychopathology, but work to increase happiness and life satisfaction as well.

COMPASSION-FOCUSED THERAPY

The development of CFT (Gilbert, 2009b, 2010a) was prompted by Gilbert's observations that shame and self-criticism were significant transdiagnostic problems for many patients. Gilbert observed that such patients, who often had early interpersonal histories that predisposed them toward self-attacking, had great difficulty generating warmth and kindness toward themselves, and often seemed somewhat unphased by traditional cognitive and behavioral interventions. For example, such patients reported that they could understand the logic of alternative, evidence-based thoughts, but did not experience affective change as a result (Gilbert, 2009b). In seeking to understand and best help such patients, Gilbert has developed an integrative model that draws upon evolutionary, social, developmental, and Buddhist psychology, as well as affective neuroscience (Gilbert, 2009b), and which is consistent with cognitive-behavioral approaches. Reflecting the pervasiveness of shame and self-attacking, CFT has been applied to a diverse variety of problems, such as depression (Gilbert, 2009c), anxiety (Tirch, 2012; Welford, 2010), overeating (Goss, 2011; Goss & Allen, 2010), shyness (Henderson, 2010), trauma (Lee & James, 2012), anger (Kolts, 2012), self-confidence (Welford, 2012), and stress reduction (Cooper, 2012), as well as with diverse populations such as individuals recovering from psychosis (Laithwaite et al., 2009) and women suffering from perinatal distress (Cree, 2010).

Like MSC, CFT seeks to assist participants in developing compassion for themselves (and others) and maintains that mindfulness skills are an important part of this process. However, CFT is based in evolutionary psychology and in a model of emotion regulation that highlights the sometimes difficult fit between our evolved emotion regulation systems; higher-order cognitive capacities for reasoning, rumination, and imagery; and the difficulties present in modern life. In CFT, the therapist works with patients to help them develop self-compassion so that they can learn to weaken and dismantle habitual patterns of self-criticism and establish new patterns of relating to themselves in ways that produce psychological states of safeness and soothing—states that will enable them to balance out threat-driven emotions and work more effectively with whatever life difficulties they find themselves faced with (Gilbert, 2010a). A primary focus of CFT is helping patients to generate, cultivate, and utilize experiences of inner warmth and compassion directed toward themselves and others.

Psychoeducation and Emotion Regulation in CFT

In the first stages of CFT, the patient is oriented to a model of emotional functioning drawn from evolutionary psychology and basic affective neuroscience. The complex world of human emotion is presented to patients via a somewhat simplified model depicting three emotion regulation systems, as described earlier. Patients learn how these emotion regulation systems evolved for three purposes: one designed to detect and respond to threats; one designed to organize us around a drive to pursue vital resources such as food, sexual partners, and pleasurable experiences; and one that is associated with feelings of safeness, comfort, and content (Gilbert 2009b, 2010a). Patients learn about these systems, and learn about the different ways they tend to organize the mind, with each involving different physiological experiences as well as patterns of attention, thinking and reasoning, motivation, and behavioral outputs (see Figure 8.1).

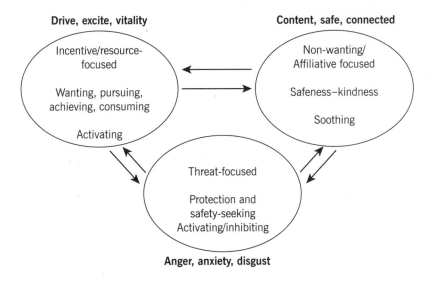

Drive, excite, vitality

Incentive/resource-focused

Wanting, pursuing, achieving, consuming

Activating

Content, safe, connected

Non-wanting/ Affiliative focused

Safeness–kindness

Soothing

Threat-focused

Protection and safety-seeking Activating/inhibiting

Anger, anxiety, disgust

FIGURE 8.1. Three types of emotion-regulation systems.

In CFT, patients learn that these emotion regulation systems evolved over millions of years in response to environmental and social demands that required our evolutionarily successful ancestors to defend themselves against predators and other threats; to acquire resources and mates; to jockey for social status; and, in the case of the safeness/soothing system, to nurture and care for helpless young, and receive nurturing and caring from others in return. Learning about these systems is designed to help patients experience their difficult, threat-based emotions not as personal flaws, but as the products of systems in their brains that evolved to protect them, but are in many cases ill-equipped to do so today, in the modern world. Patients begin to understand why it is that they can have such difficult-to-manage emotions, and learn that it is not their fault that they have them. The basis for compassion in CFT is the observation that human life is often difficult, with much of human suffering being based in the interaction of these powerful, evolved brain systems and social learning histories that we neither chose nor designed.

Compassion and Our "Old Brain"–"New Brain" Conflicts

Relatedly, CFT also educates patients about the dynamics of how certain emotions play out in the brain, highlighting the difficult ways that "old-brain"-based emotional response systems can interact with "new-brain" patterns of rumination and symbolic/representational thinking. Although the terms "old brain" and "new brain" drastically oversimplify the complex relationships among different aspects of our neural networks, they have a simplicity and a face validity that can be helpful in a clinical context. In this way, when CFT therapists begin their psychoeducation, they often refer to the "old brain," and are referring to neural structures that are much older than human beings in evolutionary terms. These are aspects of our brains and behaviors that we share with animals that are much older in evolutionary terms, such as early mammals or even reptiles. For example, the deeper brain systems involving the amygdala, sometimes known as the "fight–flight–freeze" system, which is associated with detecting and responding to threats, may be described as our "old brain." This system may be at once very powerful but not always very "wise." The "old brain" involves many behaviors, social motivations, responses, and emotions we share with other animals: being territorial, having conflicts and aggressive interactions, belonging to groups, forming alliances, experiencing sexual desires, looking after offspring—and, crucially, responding to affection and affiliation with calming. So, the idea is to help people gain clear insight into the fact that these motivational and emotional systems have been built for us, *not* by us. We simply "find ourselves here" with a mind that has these kinds of patterns of action (Gilbert, 2009a).

Next, CFT therapists explore the problems human beings have that relate to their evolved *"new" thinking brain*. Unfortunately, our evolved capacity for "thinking" creates problems as well as benefits. Around 2 million years ago human beings began to develop a whole range of cognitive abilities for imagination, reasoning, reflecting, anticipating, and developing a sense of self. Research suggests that these mental abilities may be based on the way that human beings began to derive relations among stimuli in our environment (Torneke, 2010). For human beings, a "combination of our genetically evolved capacity and a history of reinforcement by a social community" (Hayes, Strosahl, & Wilson, 2011, p. 360) has resulted in the range of what CFT refers to as *new brain psychology*: capacities for language use, symbolic understanding, problem solving, and elaboration of learning through cognition.

One of the core principles in CFT is understanding the way these new brain competencies link into, stimulate, and are stimulated by old brain motivation and emotional systems. While emotions may emerge from preverbal, *old brain* evolutionary response patterns, the human experience of emotion is expressed and derived from our cognitive and verbal behaviors, which are shaped by social contexts, and involve our *new brain* capacities. In CFT, therapists view the interaction of hardwired, prebirth-determined, emotional and motivational responding with *new brain* cognitive abilities as a part of the source of much human suffering. Take an intelligent mind and fuel it with tribal vengeance and you can end up with horrendous atrocities and nuclear weapons. Equally, take a mind with new brain competencies and link these into motivational systems that are concerned with caring and helping others and one finds the sources of compassion (Gilbert, 2009b).

While capable of powerfully organizing various aspects of mental activity around defending us from perceived dangers—producing threat-focused attention, motivation, bodily sensations, ruminations, and imagery—"old brain" emotional systems also are often not very good at distinguishing legitimate threats in the outside world from those manufactured in the frontal cortex, such as self-critical ruminative thoughts and recurrent trauma imagery. The evolutionarily designed organization of our brains, wherein old brain motivations and emotions can be reciprocally triggering with new brain capacities for symbolic thought can produce a difficult feedback loop in which the emotional threat centers are interacting with both higher-order (rumination, imagery) and lower-order (physical sensations) brain centers in ways that produce the very stimuli that then function to fuel the continued activation of the emotional threat response.

This old-brain/new-brain loop dynamic in some ways mirrors the classic cognitive-behavioral description of the way that thoughts, emotions, and behavior can interact to produce self-perpetuating patterns of affective functioning, until something comes along to help create a shift in the system (such as cognitive restructuring or behavioral activation). Similarly, the loops of the "old" and "new" brain described by CFT also involve the process described as cognitive fusion in ACT (Hayes et al., 2011). In fusion, the ways that imaginal events can exert stimulus functions on human behavior as if they were literal events in the world, leads to our behavior being dominated by maladaptive attempts to avoid or overcontrol difficult emotions.

A key message of CFT is just how much in life is not of our own choosing and is not our fault. This is not just an intellectual point. Apprehending just how much of who we are and what we do is not our fault but is designed to help patients to dis-identify from their tendency to

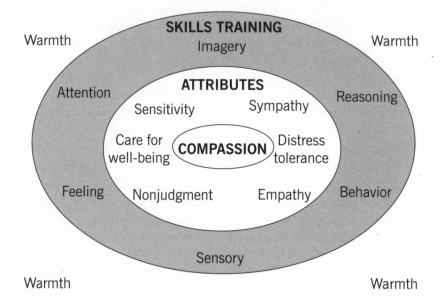

FIGURE 8.2. Multimodal compassionate mind training. From Gilbert (2009a). Used with permission from Little, Brown Book Group.

blame and shame themselves, and to activate the warmth, understanding, and loving kindness that accompany our secure attachment system and affiliative emotions.

The CFT therapist helps the patient develop this understanding through a combination of guided discovery, psychoeducation, imagery training, and other behavioral techniques. This active training of the compassionate mind is aimed at paving the way for the development of a deep compassion for themselves and others. In this way, we can perhaps see CFT as activating similar processes as elaborated in Neff's conception of common humanity, outlining the commonality of the suffering inherent to human experience.

The Development of the Compassionate Self

In CFT, compassion is operationalized in terms of specific attributes and in the skills used to develop them, depicted in Figure 8.2.

This operationalization of compassion involves the cultivation of attributes designed to assist the patient in bringing a warm sensitivity and caregiving mentality to him- or herself and his or her difficulties, as well as to endure and work with emotional discomfort. Skills training is multimodal, targets the domains historically associated with CBT (reasoning, behavior, emotion), and utilizes many techniques that will be familiar to the CBT therapist such as problem solving, examining evidence, thought work to reduce rumination, and graduated exposure (Gilbert, 2009b). As we experienced in the Compassionate Self practice, CFT makes use of imagery work and attention training that harkens to Buddhist mind-training approaches, designed to help the individual develop compassion and warmth for themselves and others. Ultimately, the goal of CFT is to assist the patient in manifesting the attributes of compassion through the cultivation of the compassionate self, which is targeted by numerous exercises.

Mindfulness in CFT

While the practice of mindfulness meditation may receive relatively less focus in CFT than in MSC, mindfulness is seen as a core competency that patients will need to develop in learning to work compassionately with their emotions. In particular, CFT emphasizes the role of nonjudgmental, mindful awareness in being able to notice and work with bodily sensations, threat emotions, self-critical thoughts, and problematic rumination and imagery. For example, patients are trained to mindfully notice when thoughts, bodily sensations, or emotional experiences of a threat response emerge in them, giving them a bit of distance from the experience as well as the possibility of responding in any number of ways—with an emphasis on relating to themselves in accepting and compassionate ways. In CFT, the mindful labeling of such experiences can take the form of, "Look—there goes my threat system again! I am really feeling [anxious, angry, etc.]. What would help me to feel safe right now so I can deal with this situation in a way that isn't dictated by my threat emotions?"

Case Conceptualization in CFT

In CFT, many patient difficulties are conceptualized as being the unintended by-products of a maladaptive threat response. The idea is that, in the face of perceived internal or external threats (many of which may originate in various historical influences such as an insecure attachment history), patients will often engage in maladaptive coping efforts, which are referred to as "safety strategies" in CFT (Gilbert, 2010a). These safety strategies, which can be either reflexively avoidant or well-intentioned efforts at avoiding internal or external harms, often produce unwanted consequences that then create further suffering in the patient's life. Examples of such safety strategies can include things like experiential avoidance, aggressive acting out, self-harm, isolation, and suicidal ideation. Maintained both by short-term benefits such as relief and belief systems, such efforts are seen (and explored) as problem-solving attempts on the part of the patient that are designed to reduce the aversive threat emotions, but are flawed (high-cost, short-term) strategies, because they are entirely based in the reasoning of the threat system—which is driven by evolutionary imperatives focused on overcoming, fleeing, or avoiding threats. In helping patients to understand these dynamics, CFT seeks to help them form an emotional understanding of the connectedness between these safety strategies and early life events—seeking to deshame their understanding of both the difficult emotions and the strategies they have engaged in as they've attempted to cope with them (Gilbert, 2010a). The treatment approach utilized in CFT is focused on helping the patient move out of a threat-driven mode of processing, to stimulate emotion-regulation systems associated with feelings of safeness, and to assist them in developing skills to work directly and adaptively with problematic situations. Once this shift has been facilitated, the CFT therapist can then make use of a variety of more traditional cognitive-behavioral techniques, such as exposure, activity scheduling, thought records, and things like this.

The exercise below is an example of an imagery practice that is used in CFT to assist patients in generating feelings of safeness and comfort.

The Compassionate Safe Space

Guided Instructions

Begin by assuming an upright, dignified posture, relaxing your facial muscles, and allowing your mouth to form a warm, slight smile. Allow your breathing to slow, and spend 30 seconds or so focusing on your breath, noting the sense of slowing in your body and mind.

When you are ready, allow yourself to imagine being in a place that is comfortable and soothing to you. Imagine that in this place you are filled with a sense of safety and calm comfort. This is your place, filled with sights, sounds, and experiences that are comforting to you.

Imagine the details of this place. What do you see? Hear? Smell? Feel? Really try to form a mental experience of what it is like here. Spend a few moments (30 seconds to a minute or longer if you like) imagining what this place is like.

Are there other beings (people, animals) here? If so, imagine that they are welcoming to you, value you, and are glad you are here. Imagine that this place itself takes joy in the fact that you are here, that this place itself welcomes you, accepts you, and is happy that you are here.

Spend as long as you like imagining and exploring this safe, comforting place. If thoughts intrude or distract you, mindfully notice them as distractions (attempting not to judge them or get caught up with them), and bring your attention back to your safe place. It's okay to resist the pull of the angry thoughts, despite how urgent they may feel. This urgent quality is simply a quality of threat emotions. Don't worry—you'll go back and attend to these things later, when things feel a bit more balanced. For now, it's all right to stay in this soothing space for a bit, and to allow yourself to feel safe, comfortable, valued, and calm.

Adapted from Kolts (2012). Used with permission from Little, Brown Book Group.

Working with Cognitions in CFT

CFT tends to focus on stimulating affective responses that involve an experience of safeness and compassion, and helping patients to notice the thoughts and reasoning that naturally arise with their compassionate minds. Both aspects of cognitive reappraisal (Gilbert, 2010c) and cognitive defusion (Tirch, 2012) are used by CFT therapists; however, the emphasis remains solidly on evoking and training the experience of compassion. Incorporating Buddhist psychology's consistent classical mindfulness, CFT helps patients to change their relationship to their thoughts, accepting them as mental events rather than as fact or reality . . . and in many cases, as mental events that are the product of a hyperactivated threat or drive response. As in other mindfulness-based treatment methods, helping patients change their relationship with troubling cognitions in this way allows them to dis-identify with the thoughts, lessening their affective impact. At the same time, CFT doesn't completely ignore content. Recognizing that mindful awareness of our thoughts is very difficult to maintain constantly and that for this reason (even for those of us who work consistently to cultivate mindfulness in our lives) our thoughts often will impact our emotional states, CFT emphasizes helping patients to cultivate specific types of thoughts—thoughts that are compassionate and kind to oneself and others. Patients are taught to observe the differences between angry, threat-driven thinking and compassionate thinking, as reflected in Table 8.1.

TABLE 8.1. Angry versus Compassionate Thinking

Angry thinking	Compassionate thinking
Narrowly focuses on the threat or object of our anger.	Broad; considers many factors in understanding the situation.
Inflexible and ruminative.	Flexible; problem-solves.
Activates our threat system; fuels anger.	Activates our safeness system; helps us to feel comfortable and at peace.
Directs hostility toward others and ourselves.	Directs kindness toward others and ourselves.
Judgmental and critical.	Noncritical and empathic.
Focuses on dominating or punishing.	Focuses on helping ourselves and others, finding solutions that benefit everyone and harm no one.

Note. Reprinted with permission from Little, Brown Book Group from Kolts, R. (2012) *The Compassionate Mind Approach for Working with Your Anger.*

After learning about compassionate thinking, patients then are prompted to identify their own threat-driven thoughts, and then to generate compassionate alternatives (see Table 8.2).

In generating compassionate alternatives, there is a focus on evidence gathering, but unlike some classic cognitive-restructuring interventions, thought work in CFT is not really focused on disputing the content of the unhelpful, threat-driven cognitions. Rather, these cognitions are simply (and mindfully) observed as understandable products of the threat system, and new, more helpful ways of thinking are generated—the goal being to cultivate cognitions that are both accurate and that assist the individual in generating feelings of safeness and warmth toward themselves and others, and in initiating positive coping efforts. Over time, patients work to develop new, compassionate ways of thinking into habitual patterns that can come to replace the older, unhelpful patterns of thoughts, slowly weakening the hold of the threat system on the individual's thinking habits. In this way, thought work in CFT seeks to accomplish two goals: helping patients to relate to all of their thoughts with compassion and mindful acceptance, and specifically cultivating habits of compassionate thinking that will be helpful in balancing their emotions and work with life challenges (Kolts, 2012).

TABLE 8.2. Compassionate Thinking Example

Angry thoughts	Compassionate thoughts
"Joshua [son] is lazy with no concern for his future."	"I'm frustrated with the choices he's making because I want him to have a good life. Maybe I could express my concerns as a caring parent more rather than just as anger. Maybe I could ask him what his plan is."
"He takes all my help for granted. He doesn't appreciate anything I've done for him."	"I feel like he disregards my advice because he makes choices that I don't agree with. Parents often want their children to do the things they think are best—but sometimes children just need to find their own way in the world. Maybe this is more about that. I could explore this with him. Just because he doesn't do everything I ask doesn't mean that he doesn't appreciate what I've done for him."
"My coworkers must think that I'm a terrible parent. I've failed at the most important task of my life."	"There is no evidence I have failed. My son is a kind person—a decent human being—even if he does sometimes struggle in terms of knowing what he wants to do. My coworkers brag about their own kids because they are proud of them—it doesn't mean they are looking down on Josh and me. It's hard to watch Josh make different choices than I would like, but they are his choices to make. I can't control him, and I want him to be his own man. Things could be a lot worse."
"First he jumps from major to major, and now he settles on *art*. He'll never have a good job, and he'll probably be dependent on me his entire life. My parents would have cut me off a long time ago!"	"I care about Josh, and I'm worried about him being able to support himself as an artist. In some ways, though, I admire his courage in choosing to pursue something that makes him happy, rather than just rushing through school like my parents pushed me to. I've made a good living, but I often hate my job—I may actually be *jealous* of Josh! Maybe I should worry less about him and focus more on *my own life*."

Note. From Kolts (2012). Reprinted with permission from Little, Brown Book Group.

Supporting Evidence

While the sheer breadth and diversity of the CFT approach has presented challenges for its empirical evaluation, CFT is the subject of an evolving body of research. In addition to the previously discussed studies that have documented the beneficial effects of self-compassion more generally, a number of studies provide initial support for specific

CFT interventions. In an early clinical trial involving a group of people attending a day hospital with chronic mental health problems, Gilbert and Procter (2006) found that CFT significantly reduced self-criticism, shame, sense of inferiority, depression, and anxiety. In a randomized controlled trial using CFT for people with psychotic disorders, Braehler and colleagues (2012) found significant clinical improvement and increases in compassion, as well as high levels of tolerability and low attrition, as compared to a treatment as usual condition. In a clinical trial, Laithwaite and colleagues (2010) found significant effects for depression, self-esteem, and an improvement in sense of self compared to others in a sample of patients in recovery from psychosis in a forensic mental health setting. In other outcome research, CFT has been found to be significantly effective for the treatment of personality disorders (Lucre & Corten, 2013), eating disorders (Gale, Gilbert, Read, & Goss, 2012), and heterogeneous mental health problems in people presenting to community mental health teams (Judge, Cleghorn, McEwan, & Gilbert, 2012). As CFT is more widely disseminated, and a growing number of clinicians and researchers become skilled in their understanding of its methods and philosophy, increasing outcome research is likely to further test the model, leading to innovation and change. While CFT-specific approaches need further empirical support, including further randomized clinical trial data, the initial research examining CFT suggest its value as a viable approach for helping individuals for whom shame and self-criticism play a significant role.

SUMMARY

For better than two millennia, Buddhism has championed the cultivation of compassion as a primary means for training the mind to free oneself and others from suffering. A growing body of evidence increasingly suggests that cultivating compassion and loving-kindness for oneself and others yields significant emotional benefits, and psychology has begun to follow suit. Recent cognitive-behavioral models such as MSCT and CFT provide clinicians with ways to utilize compassion-based interventions in the therapy room, particularly in the case of patients who struggle with shame and self-hatred.

Deeper into the Middle Path Evidence Base

I believe that spirituality and science are
complementary but different investigative approaches
with the same goal of seeking the truth. . . . In this,
there is much each may learn from the other, and
together they may contribute to expanding the horizon
of human knowledge and wisdom.
—DALAI LAMA (2005, p. 216)

RESEARCH AND THE MIDDLE PATH INTERVENTION

Throughout this book, we have drawn from a great many studies and
resources in the psychological sciences that support the efficacy of elements of Buddhist psychology in the alleviation of human suffering,
particularly as applied within CBT. While Buddhist psychology's history is distinct from the conceptual roots of Western psychology and
science, it is clear that both Buddhist psychology and CBT provide us
with a complimentary view of many of the core concerns and pursuits of
cognitive-behavioral science. For example, both concern developing an
understanding of the nature of the mind and of human suffering. Furthermore, both investigate the limits of human potential for growth, and
both seek out effective methods to promote psychological change and
well-being. Many scientists, researchers, religious leaders, and psychologists agree that an exploration of the relationship and dialogue between

Buddhism and modern sciences may foster more effective approaches to this common pursuit (Dalai Lama, 1991; Kang & Whittingham, 2010). The ensuing body of research spans several schools of science, psychology, medicine, and neurobiology (Lopez, 2009).

Given the nature of applied Buddhist psychology as an eight-component program for liberation from suffering, it makes sense to relate the Noble Eightfold Path to the scientific literature directly. What follows is a selection of the research on Buddhist psychology and CBT, intended as a map to help you navigate the empirical research base. To date, there is no research on a comprehensive approach to Buddhist psychology-focused CBT, nor does there exist an all-inclusive, evidence-based, secularized Middle Path intervention. However, this integrative analysis of select Buddhist psychology-related research (including Buddhist psychology-based meditation, compassion, and mindfulness training) intends to be comparative, not declarative, in nature.

The Eightfold Path or the Middle Path intervention aims to be a route toward healthy living, freeing oneself from the "cycle of suffering" (*samsara*). There are several interrelated practices and processes involved in each of these steps. Thus, in this chapter, we explore the recent psychological research on Buddhist psychology-informed treatments, processes, and practices as they specifically relate to each of the components of the Middle Path. The sections below discuss modern research as it applies to adaptive and healthy speech, action, livelihood, effort, concentration, mindfulness, thought, and understanding. Importantly, we can notice that a great deal of the research supporting the various elements of the Middle Path are derived from the body of literature that explores "mindfulness training." As Kabat-Zinn (2009) has repeatedly noted, the development of such training in the West initially used the term "mindfulness" as an umbrella term to describe the coming together of many elements of the *dharma*, in a way that could be presented as secular, and as free from cultural baggage as possible. It is not surprising, then, that when we seek out the scientific support for each of the elements in the Eightfold Path, it will be found in research that is described as studying "mindfulness."

HEALTHY SPEECH

As established in Chapter 2, *Healthy Speech* refers specifically to speaking with honesty, clarity, and skill; and generally refers to more effective forms of communication. Buddhist psychology interventions, such as those that emphasize compassion and mindfulness, may help us improve the way we communicate and relate to others (Hartnett, 2010) and to ourselves. Speech can be considered as an interpersonal and intrapersonal process—and like other complex, multivariable, context-dependent psychological processes, it is a challenge to measure.

There is a small but growing body of research examining direct behavioral changes in social speech and self-speech in relation to Buddhist psychology-based training that includes research on meditation, mindfulness-based training, and compassion-based interventions. A number of authors have observed the logical link between mindfulness training and effective communication. Wood (2004) proposed mindfulness training as a contributor to more effective communication and less reactive and defensive behaviors in social situations. Similarly, Huston and colleagues (2011) suggested that mindfulness in combination with communication training can increase interpersonal and intrapersonal self-awareness, self-regulation, resilience, flexibility, and empathy. When added to an introductory course in communication for students, mindfulness training was associated with their increases in positive reappraisal compared to individuals who received the communication course without the mindfulness component, suggesting the potential of mindfulness to reduce negative reactivity in interpersonal exchanges.

Both dispositional mindfulness, defined as our innate and untrained capacity for mindfulness, and mindfulness training are associated with effective communication and reduced conflict in relationships (Barnes, Brown, Krusemark, Campbell, & Rogge, 2007; Wachs & Cordova, 2007). For instance, individuals reporting higher levels of dispositional mindfulness engaged in less hostility and verbal aggression within their romantic relationships than did individuals lower in self-reported mindfulness (Barnes et al., 2007). Furthermore, this study using a correlational, short-term longitudinal design revealed that individuals higher in mindfulness reported higher levels of satisfaction with their romantic relationships. The authors also reported evidence of a significant role for mindfulness in enhancing adaptive responses to relationship stress. In regard to relationship conflict, this research also found dispositional mindfulness was related to lower levels of negative emotion, more positive perceptions of the relationship and the partner and after a conflictual exchange, and that state-related mindfulness was related to better communication quality during the discussion (Barnes et al., 2007). Wachs and Cordova (2007) conducted research with married couples and found that the association between mindfulness and marital qual-ity was mediated by skillful or effective behavioral repertoires, in par-ticular, identifying and communicating emotions and the regulation of anger expression.

With regard to facilitating effective communication or *healthy speech*, mindfulness has also been associated with less hostility and defensiveness (Lakey, Kernis, Heppner, & Lance, 2008). For example, individuals who completed mindfulness-based training displayed less aggression after receiving social rejection feedback than individuals who did not receive the training (Heppner et al., 2008). Furthermore, dis-positional mindfulness has also been correlated with higher authentic-ity and lower levels of verbal defensiveness (Lakey et al., 2008). In this study, participants who completed self-reported measures of authentic-ity and dispositional mindfulness subsequently completed an assessment of defensive verbal behavior in which their responses to potentially self-threatening stimuli were rated for openness and honesty versus defen-siveness. These researchers found a positive correlation between authen-ticity and mindfulness, with higher scores on each being related to lower levels of verbal defensiveness. Additional analysis revealed that mindful-ness mediated the observed relationship between authenticity and verbal defensiveness (Lakey et al., 2008).

Compassion-based training and LKM have both been examined in regard to their relationship with effective communication and values-based interpersonal responding. For example, in a case study of a group LKM-based training, patients experiencing psychosis attended a weekly LKM group for 6 weeks and a follow-up review session occurring 6 weeks after the termination of the group. Each of the sessions included discussion, skills teaching, and practice. The authors report that these individuals exhibited a reduction in negative symptoms, particularly a reduction in the experiences of emotional blunting, after completing the training (Johnson et al., 2009). Given the observed reduction of negative symptoms in this study, there is a distinct possibility that compassion-based interventions may increase social responding and communication with individuals experiencing psychosis. Other research suggests that LKM may activate areas of the brain associated with empathy toward others, which could play a role in the fostering of social responding and enhancement of relationships (Lutz et al., 2008).

Interpersonal behavior changes were also found after compas-sion training in a study regarding the use of punishment. Condon and

DeSteno (2011) found that formal compassion training reduced partici-pants' tendency to engage in punishment of others. This study exam-ined how the experience of compassion toward one person might reduce punishment directed at another person. In a staged-interaction design in which one individual cheats to earn higher compensation than others that resulted in heightened third-party punishment being directed at the cheater, this study found that punishment of the cheater was nonexistent in those participants who received compassion training toward a sepa-rate individual, despite the cheater's clear intention and lack of remorse. Furthermore, the degree of compassion participants reported directly mediated the reduction in punishment behaviors for other individuals (Condon & DeSteno, 2011).

As we have discussed, shame-based criticism has negative effects on motivation, is related to depression, and generally increases anxiety and a sense of hopelessness (Gilbert, Baldwin, Irons, Baccus, & Palmer, 2006; Longe et al., 2010). Shame-based self-criticism has a negative impact upon responses to treatment for major depression (Marshall, Zuroff, McBride, & Bagby, 2008; Rector et al., 2000). We might even consider shaming communications directed toward the self and others as an example of one of the most *unhelpful* forms of speech. Cognitive-behavioral interventions drawing from Buddhist psychology, most nota-bly CFT, have been shown to be effective in increasing compassionate correction and buffering against the negative impacts of shame-based self-criticism (Gilbert & Procter, 2006). For example, in a pilot study conducted by Gilbert and Procter (2006), a small number of patients who suffered from depression and were high in shame and self-criticism received compassionate mind training in a group setting, where they learned to foster compassionate attitudes and increase awareness of self-critical thoughts as ineffective mental habits. Postintervention results revealed reductions in anxiety, depression, shame, self-criticism, sense of inferiority, and submissive behavior.

Self-compassion training has also demonstrated similar results (Neff, 2003b; Neff et al., 2007). Other research and use of Buddhist psychology-based interventions and implications for right speech include the application of ACT to racial prejudice with promising results (Lillis & Hayes, 2007), the use of mindfulness-based interper-sonal effectiveness skills (Linehan, 1993a), and the use of mindfulness-informed communication in hospice or palliative care settings (Vil-ligran et al., 2010).

HEALTHY ACTION

The concept of *Healthy Action*, as introduced in Chapter 3 as the second component of *Adaptive Conduct*, involves behaving in ways that are kind, helpful, and ultimately promote the well-being of self and others, and refraining from behaviors that cause harm. It is about acting in skillful and valued ways that do not harm the self or others on their path. Specific Buddhist psychology-based interventions may facilitate a deeper understanding of one's emotions, and, in turn, a clearer sense of what really matters: one's personal values, and those responses or behaviors that embody or prove effective in pursuing one's values. Furthermore, as we have discussed earlier, flexible, values-based responses to present moment consequences have been found to correlate with a number of positive psychological outcomes in the behavioral science literature (Hayes, 2008b). In fact, recent research indicates that commitment to a purpose in life and engagement in those related behaviors provides daily enrichment and increased reports of well-being in individuals with social anxiety disorder (SAD) (Kashdan & McNight, 2013).

Values clarification and improved behavioral self-regulation may be two additional avenues through which acceptance, mindfulness, and compassion-based training enhance *healthy action* and improve psychological well-being (Wallace & Shapiro, 2006) and psychological flexibility (Fledderus, Bohlmeijer, Smit, & Westerhof, 2010). Dispositional mindfulness has been associated with self-reports of more engagement in values-based behaviors and pursuits (Brown & Ryan, 2003). Furthermore, values clarification was found to partially mediate the observed relationship between higher levels of mindfulness and decreased psychological distress in a sample of MBSR participants (Carmody, Baer, Lykins, & Olendzki, 2009). Mindfulness has also been correlated with the ability to continue in goal-directed behavior in the presence of negative affect (Baer, Smith, Hopkins, Krietemeyer, & Taney, 2006). The research on *healthy action* and Buddhist psychology can be divided into behaviors related to valued areas of living: relationships, wellness, play/creativity, and work (which will be covered in the review of the research related to *Adaptive Livelihood*).

Healthy Action and Relationships

Considering prosocial behavior as a primary example of *healthy action*, we find a number of strands of research that support the use of Buddhist psychology-inspired interventions as effective in supporting the ability of individuals to experience interpersonal connectedness and to behave effectively and helpfully in relation to others. Research has linked mindfulness and various forms of compassion training to relationship satisfaction and enhancement (Carson, Carson, Gil, & Baucom, 2004); empathy and perspective taking (Birnie, Speca, & Carlson, 2010); and self-reported adaptive socioemotional functioning (Sahdra et al., 2011).

In an empirical study of mindfulness and relationship satisfaction and enhancement, Carson and his colleagues (2004) conducted a randomized controlled study to test the efficacy of an MBSR-based couple program, mindfulness-based relationship enhancement, for relatively nondistressed romantic couples. Mindfulness was linked with enriched current relationship functioning and improved individual psychological well-being across a wide range of indicators. The findings indicate that the intervention positively impacted levels of relationship satisfaction, autonomy, relatedness, closeness, acceptance of one another, and relationship distress. Additionally, participants also reported beneficial changes in optimism, spirituality, relaxation, and psychological distress, with gains maintained at 3-month follow-up. Furthermore, participants who practiced mindfulness more frequently revealed superior outcomes compared to those who practiced less, and analyses of daily diary measures showed greater mindfulness practice on a given day was related to several consecutive days of improved relationship happiness, stress-coping efficacy, and reduced levels of relationship stress and overall stress (Carson et al., 2004). Relatedly, mindfulness has also been correlated with the ability to act with awareness in social situations (Dekeyser, Raes, Leijssen, Leyson, & Dewulf, 2008).

Training in certain contemplative practices is believed to cultivate prosocial behavior, a contention that is supported by a growing body of empirical work. For example, Kremeny and colleagues (2012) provide an example of how Buddhist psychology-inspired meditation techniques can be combined with emotional skills training to facilitate prosocial behavior and an enhanced ability to respond helpfully to suffering. These researchers utilized an 8-week training program (42 hours total) involving an integration of didactics, discussion, practice of meditation (concentration meditation, mindfulness meditation, and directive practices that focused on empathy, perspective taking, and compassion), and emotion-based skills learning (instruction in understanding the components of emotions and their antecedents and consequences, recognizing emotions in self and others and the connections between emotion and cognition, and recognizing emotional patterns in one's self). The results indicate that this intervention also enhanced prosocial responding, including compassion, and reduced negative social responding. Participants involved in the training revealed a greater facility in the recognition of emotional facial expressions and, when presented with an image of a suffering individual, were more likely than controls to respond with compassion-based rather than disgust-based semantic responses. In an additional task, referred to as the "provocative marital interaction task," individuals in the training group were significantly less likely to engage in hostile behavior compared to individuals in the control group. Finally, the training group appeared less susceptible to responding with enhanced negative behavior in regards to the task of resolving a challenging relationship problem. The authors conclude that certain prosocial responses can be improved and destructive emotional responses can be reduced with a meditation-based intervention.

Similarly, empirical research has linked LKM with increased feelings of social connectedness and positive affect toward strangers (Hutcherson, Seppala, & Gross, 2008). In this study, the researcher used a brief LKM exercise to examine social connection toward strangers. Compared with a matched control task, a few minutes of LKM increased reported feelings of social connection and positivity toward novel individuals.

Additionally, neuropsychological studies have demonstrated that compassion induction and training is associated with activation in regions of the brain implicated in prosocial motivation and feelings of empathy (Engström & Söderfeldt, 2010; Kim et al., 2011). Furthermore, neuroimaging research reveals self-compassion training to be associated with neuronal activity akin to that of empathy for others (Longe et al., 2010).

With regard to compassion, one university-based research project examined the effects of first-semester college students' goals on changes in social support and trust over a semester and weekly relationship experiences. They found that having more compassionate goals was associated with feeling socially connected, a belief in mutual caring, feeling supported, and trust among first-semester college students (Crocker & Canevello, 2008). A second study revealed that more compassionate goals predicted increased social support through both interpersonal processes and intrapersonal processes. Analyses of roommate pairs indicated that participants' average levels of compassionate and self-image goals were associated with their roommates' reports of both the support received from and given to the participants. The participants who had higher compassionate goals had consistently higher roommate reports of both given and received social support; however, this result only seemed to be the case for participants who were low in self-image goals (Crocker & Canevello, 2008). This study supports the Buddhist psychology contention that compassion facilitates skillful engagement with others, while ego-based self-preoccupation inhibits our ability to connect, even if our goals are good ones.

While self-image goals may not help us to skillfully connect with others, there is some evidence suggesting that self-compassion can. Baker and McNulty (2011) examined the association of self-compassion to relationship maintenance processes and behaviors (including interpersonal motivation to correct mistakes, effective problem solving, and adaptive behaviors) and relationship satisfaction in men and women. This study revealed positive associations between self-compassion and relationship maintenance and satisfaction in both women and men. However, in men, these associations appeared to apply only in the instance of conscientiousness. This finding is important in highlighting an interpersonal dimension to self-compassion, suggesting that the ability to direct compassion to oneself can significantly impact upon one's relationships with others (Baker & McNulty, 2011).

Healthy Action and Wellness

Practices rooted in Buddhist psychology have also been shown to be significantly related to adaptive psychological functioning and behavioral change. Increasing evidence suggests that these practices have a positive impact on prevention and recovery in a wide range of medical and psychological treatment contexts, and in the treatment of a range of disorders involving physiological and behavioral responses to stress as well as behaviors related to prevention morbidity and mortality (Alexander, Robinson, Orme-Johnson, Schneider, & Walton, 1994). For example, stress-related physiological changes associated with Buddhist psychology practices include decreased cortisol levels (Carlson, Speca, Faris, & Patel, 2007; Pace et al., 2009); decreased breathing rate (Lazar et al., 2000, 2005); decreased skin conductance response (Astin, 1997; Tang et al., 2009); lowered oxygen and carbon dioxide consumption (Young & Taylor, 1998); decreased heart rate (Zeidan, Johnson, Gordon, &

Goolkasian, 2010); and decreased blood pressure (de la Fuente, Franco, & Salvador, 2010).

One way that Buddhist practice might improve wellness is through enhancing motivation about self-care and healthy behaviors. A web-based survey of 886 Buddhist respondents (82% of whom were U.S. residents) inquired about individual religious practices and beliefs, health history, and health-related behaviors (Wiist, Sullivan, George, & Wayment, 2012). Results indicated that 68% of the respondents reported their health as "very good" or "excellent." Another interesting finding in this study revealed that a 1-point increase on the Buddhist Devoutness Index used in the survey was associated with an 11% increase in the chance of being in good to excellent health and a 15% increase in the chance of being a nonsmoker (Wiist et al., 2012).

Mindfulness has specifically been related to self-regulation as well as to enhanced well-being. For example, one study examined the results of self-reported mindfulness, utilizing various measures relating to self-regulation of sleep and a comprehensive measure of emotional, psychological, and social well-being in undergraduate students ($N = 334$). The findings indicated that mindfulness predicted well-being both directly and indirectly through its association with self-regulation of sleep. Similarly, with regard to diet and exercise, research has revealed that the degree of mindfulness in everyday life is predictive of the amount of fruit and vegetable intake, fat intake (only for men), physical activity, and perceived self-efficacy (Gilbert & Waltz, 2010).

Preliminary evidence also suggests that mindfulness-based treatments can facilitate decreases in dysregulated problem behaviors such as gambling (Lakey, Campbell, Brown, & Goodie, 2007; Toneatto, Vettese, & Nguyen, 2007) and substance use (Bowen et al., 2009; Bowen, Chawla, & Marlatt, 2011; Wupperman et al., 2012). One example is a pilot study of mindfulness and modification therapy (MMT) for women who had recently been arrested for domestic violence and met criteria for alcohol abuse or dependence and aggression ($N = 14$). In this study, participants participated in a treatment program involving 12 weekly individual sessions (an initial 90-minute session followed by eleven 60-minute sessions). With a retention rate of 93%, the study's pre–post comparisons revealed significant decreases in alcohol use, drug use, and aggression among study participants (Wupperman et al., 2012).

Self-compassion has also been proposed as a useful intervention with a variety of illnesses and disorders (Terry & Leary, 2011). For instance, Kelly, Zuroff, Foa, and Gilbert (2010) examined the use of compassionate imagery and self-talk for smoking cessation interventions. The results of this study implicated self-compassion techniques as helping to facilitate the reduction of smoking behaviors more quickly than the self-monitoring group, but at the same rate as self-energizing and self-controlling groups. Furthermore, the results of this study seemed to indicate that self-compassion interventions are particularly potent for specific types of patients; the effects of the self-compassion training depended on participants who had higher levels of self-criticism, lower readiness to change, and more vivid imagery during intervention exercises. These results are heartening in that they point to a potential role of self-compassion interventions in helping individuals who may be less responsive to other methods by addressing self-critical handicapping and increasing motivation to change.

In regard to psychological health and treatment, the research on Buddhist psychology-based interventions is growing almost by the day. For a review of the effects of mindfulness and psychological health, see Keng and colleagues (2011) and Sedlmeier and colleagues (2012). A full review of this literature is beyond the scope of this book, so we'll highlight some findings here that we think are important in understanding the breadth and depth of the potential applications of Buddhist psychology in the service of psychological health.

One of the largest areas of growth has been in the treatment of depression and anxiety. Exposure therapy interventions have long been considered the "gold standard" in the effective reduction of fear-based responding and experiential avoidance (Chambless & Ollendick, 2001). The benefits of health-related behavior changes observed following Buddhist psychology-based exposure is quite apparent in those treatments and studies for anxiety disorders (Greeson & Brantley, 2009), and there is growing evidence for these applications and reduction in avoidance behaviors in the treatment of generalized anxiety disorder (GAD) (Roemer et al., 2008), obsessive–compulsive disorder (OCD) (Hale, Strauss, & Taylor, 2013; Hannan & Tolin, 2005), and PTSD (Kimbrough, Magyari, Langenberg, Chesney, & Berman, 2010).

In traditional exposure treatment, patients are exposed to their feared stimuli and refrained from engaging in their safety behaviors (typically various methods of experiential avoidance of both internal and external stimuli). Clinical research has revealed that the benefits of exposure are hindered by the use of such safety behaviors (Lovibond,

Mitchell, Minard, Brady, & Menzies, 2009; Salkovskis, Clark, Hackmann, Wells, & Gelder, 1999; Wells, 1995).

Preliminary evidence suggests that Buddhist psychology training such as mindfulness and compassion-based practices can be effective in regards to exposure and can promote significant changes of previously held stimulus–response patterns (Treanor, 2011). For example, mindfulness is believed to play a major role in the shift and reduction in the practitioner's self-perceived reactivity and the facilitation of exposure (Hölzel et al., 2011). The learning that transpires in mindful experience is akin to the learning that occurs with exposure in traditional CBT approaches, in that the practitioner learns that unpleasant feelings or stimuli come and go, leaving a sense of well-being or safety (Öst, 1997). Therefore, through the nature and qualities of mindfulness such as an open awareness, acceptance, and nonattachment, mindfulness practice can potentially minimize the use of safety behaviors and maximize the effects of exposure to previously avoided and feared stimuli. The capacity to remain psychologically present in the face of internal experiences is a core quality of mindfulness, embodied in the "non-reactivity to inner experience" subscale of the Five Facets of Mindfulness Questionnaire. Carmody and Baer (2008) found that study participants upon completion of an MBSR course reported significant increases with large effect sizes on the nonreactivity to inner experiences scale. Additionally, another study found that participants who completed an MBSR training course revealed significant pre- to postintervention increases in their willingness to experience exposure to unpleasant experiences (Carmody et al., 2009). Nonreactivity and exposure processes appear to be crucial players in the stress-reduction effects of mindfulness and in decreased perceived stress scores (Carmody & Baer, 2008; Chang et al., 2004).

HEALTHY LIVELIHOOD

As you may remember from Chapter 3, *Right Livelihood* extends from the concept of Right Action to emphasize how we embody action in our work and livelihood. Research on mindfulness and compassion-based interventions have promising implications in creating contexts for change in the area of *healthy livelihood* and the facilitation of more effective working relationships and work environments (Atkins & Parker, 2011).

Compassion is seen as having a positive influence in the workplace (Kanov et al., 2004). There is growing interest and research in the area of positive organizational psychology (Bernstein, 2003). This research focuses on organizational processes as a whole (Dutton et al., 2006), as well as on individual development (Atkins & Parker, 2011) at both the interpersonal (Kanov et al., 2004) and intrapersonal levels (Shepherd & Cardon, 2009). The focus here is on those factors that contribute to the cultivation of strengths, vitality, and thriving to allow for individual and organizational reliance, flourishing, and skillful effective functioning. One of these factors of interest is compassion (Bernstein, 2003). The emphasis in this approach stands counter to typical, more destructive, aims such as greed and competitiveness (Shepherd & Cardon, 2009). Shepherd and Cardon (2009) propose that self-compassion training might improve responding to and learning from failures in the workplace.

HEALTHY EFFORT

Traditionally in Buddhist psychology, *Mental Discipline* is taught and trained through various methods, the primary of which is meditation. Various medidation practices provide different forms of training that focus on different aspects of a meditator's attention and awareness. The intention paid to each of these mental discipline practices involves *Healthy Effort*—an intentional, willing, skillful approach requiring patience, diligence, and motivation. Whether it be in meditation or in life, *Adaptive Effort* focuses on intention and effectiveness.

A prime example of such *Healthy Effort* involves processes of acceptance. Williams and Lynn (2011) define and address the process of acceptance as it relates to both psychopathology and clinical interventions. Acceptance can be considered the process of just letting things be and experiencing them as they are, and is often included as a core component of mindfulness. The relationship between acceptance and behavior change is a nuanced one. While acceptance can be seen as the opposite of a change-focused motivation, it can also be considered as a necessary precursor—a crucial first step—toward behavior change (Germer, 2005a). Acceptance-based processes have been prominently featured in research and clinical applications such as ACT, which emphasize the role of acceptance in reducing processes of experiential avoidance. Furthermore, acceptance is one half of the "acceptance and change" dynamic present in DBT. This increasing understanding of the paradoxical nature of acceptance and change and the role of experiential avoidance in psychopathology has led to the increased use of mindfulness and other Buddhist psychology practices that emphasize full acceptance of life on life's terms.

Research on acceptance suggests that it serves a protective role in the face of situations that are perceived as stressful, negative, or threatening. Shallcross, Troy, Boland, and Mauss (2010) conducted two studies to explore the role of acceptance in shaping affective reactions to such experiences. The first of these examined the interaction between acceptance and emotional context. Female college undergraduate participants were categorized into two groups based on high or low scores on the Acceptance and Action Questionnaire (AAQ; Hayes et al., 2006). Participants viewed two film clips in order, one featuring a neutral emotional content and another with a negative emotional content, and rated their levels of negative affect after watching each clip. Results indicated that high-acceptance participants experienced lower levels of negative affect than low-acceptance participants after viewing the negative emotion context film clip, whereas no significant differences in negative affect were found in the neutral emotion context. A second, prospective study conducted an initial assessment of participant levels of acceptance and current depressive symptoms, and conducted another assessment 4 months later. This study confirmed the investigators' hypothesis that acceptance appeared to buffer individuals from the development of depressive symptoms in times of high stress and there was no relationship between acceptance and depressive symptoms found during times of low stress.

HEALTHY CONCENTRATION

Healthy Concentration goes beyond simply maintaining attentional focus. It also means being able to fully engage all of one's mental faculties as one faces the challenges of life. Concentration meditation teaches control of attentional focus and is taught to bring about a calm, composed mind that is free from the influence of emotional or environmental involvement (Nhat Hahn, 1998; Rahula, 1959/1974). Concentration meditation has been proposed to produce disinhibition of awareness processes (Colby, 1991), and can be considered a unique yet related form of mental training, distinct from mindfulness (Dunn et al., 1999). Buddhist tradition emphasizes the need for concentration meditation in order to create a tranquil mind that allows unbiased examination of the mind and self (Epstein, 1995).

Valentine and Sweet (1999) compared 19 experienced concentrative and mindfulness meditators to 32 nonmeditating controls. Those who meditated demonstrated superior performance on tests of sustained attention versus the performance of control subjects. Additionally, more experienced or long-term meditators had stronger sustained attention abilities than did short-term meditators (Valentine & Sweet, 1999). Furthermore, mindfulness meditators displayed more skillful sustained attention than concentration-based meditators when the stimulus was unexpected. However, no difference between the types of meditation was observed when the stimulus was expected (Valentine & Sweet, 1999). This research supports the long-held contention of Buddhist psychology that attentional abilities can be improved through consistent use of meditative techniques designed to develop these properties of mind. We'll discuss the processes of attention in greater detail below, in our discussion of *Healthy Mindfulness*.

HEALTHY MINDFULNESS

Healthy Mindfulness, as explored in Chapter 2, is the diligent awareness of the present moment, as it is, including bodily activities, feelings, thoughts, and motivations. Mindfulness meditation broadens awareness and trains the mind to utilize a flexible focus of awareness and attention, and can provide clarity and insight into the nature of one's consciousness and experiences (Lazar et al., 2005). Siegel (2009) has proposed nine psychological functions or processes as potential benefits of mindfulness: body regulation, attuned communication, emotional balance, fear modulation, response flexibility, insight, empathy, morality, and intuition. All of these processes except for intuition have been studied in regards to Buddhist psychology processes and demonstrate strong correlations with mindfulness. Other authors have conducted comprehensive reviews and systematic meta-analyses of the literature and evidence supporting the role of mindfulness and mindfulness-based trainings in clinical psychology (Baer, 2003; Coelho, Canter, & Ernst, 2007; Grossman,

Neimann, Schmidt, & Walach, 2004; Hoffman, Sawyer, Witt, & Oh, 2010).

Buddhist psychology considers everyone to be capable of mindfulness. For some, this quality can be found naturally within their repertoire, and for others it may be more dormant, requiring more purposeful cultivation and training. The innate capacity to inhabit this stance is described as "dispositional mindfulness" and can be considered an intrinsic characteristic, the expression and experience of which varies significantly (Bishop et al., 2004; Brown & Ryan, 2003; Carlson & Brown, 2005; Kabat-Zinn, 2003). Individual differences in dispositional mindfulness have begun to emerge in research populations with strong implications for self-regulation, psychological adjustment, and well-being (Baer, Smith, & Allen, 2004; Brown & Ryan, 2003, 2004; Reibel, Greeson, Brainard, & Rozenzweig, 2001; Shapiro & Schwartz, 2000). Dispositional mindfulness has been associated with an array of positive psychological outcomes and the facilitation of adaptive regulatory processes and effective responses to situational demands (Brown, Ryan, & Creswell, 2007). Such findings include observed correlations between dispositional mindfulness and greater unconditional self-acceptance and self-esteem (Thompson & Waltz, 2008), better attuned risk-taking decisions and judgments (Lakey et al., 2007), and lower levels of negative automatic thought frequency and perceptions of the ability to let go of such thoughts (Frewen, Evans, Maraj, Dozois, & Partridge, 2008). Dispositional mindfulness has also been associated with the ability to manage and regulate negative affect (Arch & Craske, 2006; Coffey & Hartman, 2008; Lakey et al., 2007), and is negatively correlated with measures of psychological distress. Certain facets of mindfulness have demonstrated incremental validity in the prediction of symptom levels (Baer, Smith, Hopkins, Krietemeyer, & Toney, 2006; Coffey & Hartman, 2008; Vujanovic, Zvolensky, Bernstein, Feldner, & McLeish, 2007).

The inherent capacity for mindfulness may serve to reduce vulnerability to various psychological symptoms and problems, even in the face of risk factors that would otherwise increase vulnerability to such problems (Way, Creswell, Eisenberger, & Lieberman, 2010). The research on dispositional mindfulness suggests that this process stands contrary to automatic or habitual responding and has been associated with more autonomously motivated behavior (Levesque & Brown, 2007). The case can be made that mindfulness provides an increased psychological freedom in which thoughts and feelings are viewed as impermanent, transient mental events, and it is believed that possessing the capacity for mindfulness may help in the prevention and disruption of ruminative or depressogenic thought processes (Coffey & Hartman, 2008; Teasdale, 1999).

Research on Mindfulness Training and the Four Foundations of Mindfulness

Mindfulness can be regarded as a skill set that can be cultivated through the use of various techniques or meditative traditions (Bishop et al., 2004; Davidson, 2010; Linehan, 1993b). Research on the effects of mindfulness training and mindfulness-based CBT supports its role in aiding numerous treatments and enhancing well-being. For example, mindfulness training has been shown to be effective in facilitating emotion regulation (Adele & Feldman, 2004; Hofmann et al., 2010; Leahy et al., 2011), expanding awareness or metacognitive awareness (Teasdale et al., 2002), and enhancing attentional control (Teasdale, Segal, Williams, & Mark, 1995).

As we explored earlier, mindfulness training in Buddhist psychology has four foundational components: mindfulness of the body, mindfulness of feeling, mindfulness of consciousness or thought, and mindfulness of mental products. As awareness of one's thoughts, perceptions, emotions, and how those emotions play out in the body are core aims of CBT, it follows that mindfulness training seems to have an obvious fit with CBT interventions.

Mindfulness of the body is about awareness and attunement with the tangible experience, grounding oneself in the form and function of the purely physiological. Like so many things, the body can be a source of significant suffering but also the alleviation of suffering. For example, in the traditional treatment of panic, interoceptive exposure aims to change the dysfunctional associations between somatic changes and feared responding. There is reason to believe that mindfulness training can facilitate this therapeutic process. Increased awareness of physical sensation and interoceptive perception are reported by both long-term meditation practitioners and participants in MBSR training (Carmody & Baer, 2008; Hölzel, Ott, Hempel, & Stark, 2006). In an interview-based study, seven out of 10 experienced meditators reported increased perception and awareness of physical sensations, and four of the 10 reported an increased awareness of emotion (Hölzel et al., 2006).

The second foundation is mindfulness of feeling. Buddhist teachings and modern psychology recognize both the destructive and the healing capacities of thoughts and emotions (Hayes & Feldman, 2004). Emotion regulation and mindfulness are strongly related in the psychological literature. Affect labeling is a first step in emotion regulation and has been shown to disrupt the automatic emotional responding and reduce the intensity and duration of an emotion (Lieberman et al., 2007). The "observing and noting" of affective experiences practiced in many Buddhist psychology meditative traditions parallel this process. Additionally, numerous authors have proposed affect tolerance as a result of the accepting and nonjudgmental approach to emotions that is taken in mindfulness (Bishop et al., 2004; Epstein, 1995; Hayes & Feldman, 2004; Linehan, 1993a). Buddhist psychology highlights the need to be "free from destructive emotions while at the same time seeing that such freedom comes through nonjudgmental awareness of just those emotions from which we seek freedom" (Epstein, 1995, p. 24).

The third foundation is known as mindfulness of states of mind or mindfulness of cognition, including both the state or tone of the mind and its cognitive processes. Similar to many cognitive-behavioral therapies, the focus is on noticing how direct experience can provoke cognition. This involves watching the mind transform our experience and interaction with our context into thoughts. In other words, it involves both training and observing the mechanisms of cognition at work. This practice highlights discernment, evaluations, judgments, and a degree of openness to experience.

Theorists have proposed that mindfulness interventions may promote positive adjustment by fortifying metacognitive skills (Hamilton, Kitzman, & Gutotte, 2006). Additionally, previous research has implicated dispositional mindfulness in the capacity to let go of negative thoughts and potentially increase an individual's level of cognitive flexibility (Frewen et al., 2008). The ability to engage in the nonjudgmental, unattached mode of mindfulness has been implicated in the attenuation of unwanted, maladaptive, or affect-laden preconceptions and behaviors through enhanced regulatory capabilities (Hayes & Feldman, 2004; Shapiro & Schwartz, 2000).

Essential cognitive processes involved in mindfulness include attention, awareness, and acceptance, all of which seem to have symbiotic, complex, irreducibly intertwined relationships within the nature of consciousness and one another. For example, the attention and awareness processes involved in mindfulness, such as bare attention and meta-awareness, interact to foster the present-centered, nonjudgmental, observer perspective (Nyanaponika, 1973). In regard to mindfulness, these processes work together to change the way in which one experiences the self, the world, and reality itself.

Awareness is described as the subjective observation or registration of internal and external stimuli (Brown & Ryan, 2003; Brown et al., 2007). *Vipassana* (Pali) is translated as "insight" or "clear awareness" medidation, which involves nonelaborative, open awareness toward the full spectrum of the present moment (Davis & Hayes, 2011; Gunaratana, 2002). This present-centeredness promotes a heightened awareness of one's mind, body, and environment, and allows an individual to feel unified with his or her experience and feel what it means to be fully present, evoking a fresh understanding of the self within that particular moment (Carmody & Baer, 2008; Hayes & Feldman, 2004). For example, one study found that after 9 weeks of Zen meditation practice, randomly assigned counselor students/trainees reported higher levels of self-awareness compared to nonmeditating counselor trainees (Grepmair et al., 2007).

Mindful awareness is alert and open to all that is available in a given moment and has been described as "choiceless awareness." Additionally, this receptive stance can be characterized as meta-awareness, or "awareness of awareness" (Brown & Cordon, 2009; Corcoran, Farb, Anderson, & Segal, 2010; Nyanaponika, 1973). Choiceless awareness in mindfulness involves a stripping away of attachment, preferences, reflexive responses, or interpretations of experience. This nonattachment is characterized by abandoning preconceived notions or judgments surrounding any aspect of consciousness. As we discussed earlier, attachment is viewed as a (and perhaps *the*) primary source of human suffering in Buddhist traditions. In choiceless awareness, no one object of awareness is more likely to be attended to than any other and there is no longer a distinction between the observer and the observed. As Levine (1979) so eloquently describes it: "It's like standing on a stream bank, watching all the thoughts float down stream like bubbles. And as we watch, it becomes increasingly clear that some of the bubbles are us watching the stream, that even the watcher is part of the flow, and awareness simply experiences it all" (p. 29). There are several classic guided mindfulness practices that utilize this metaphor or similar images to aid the meditator in establishing the experience and capacity for choiceless awareness.

Examples include leaves on a stream, blowing thoughts into bubbles or balloons, the mind train, and the conveyer belt (Hayes, Strosahl, & Wilson, 2011).

It may be obvious to many therapists that how we pay attention and what we pay attention to have a direct influence on our mind and our experience of reality. In regard to psychological sciences, attention is often viewed as a group of discrete subprocesses, which collectively contribute to our ability to attend to and focus on various internal or external stimuli (Treadway & Lazar, 2009). One theory of attention that is widely supported and is consistent with Buddhist psychology groups attention into three types, each involving distinct neural networks and functions (Chiesa et al., 2011). These three groups are *alerting/sustained attention*, which involves the achievement and maintenance of states of readiness or vigilance; *orienting/selective attention* that limits what perceptual input is given continued attention and what is not; and *executive/divided attention*, which monitors and distributes attention and prioritizes various thoughts, emotions, and behavioral responses (Desimone, & Duncan, 1995; Duncan, 1980; McDowd, 2007; Posner & Peterson, 1990; Posner & Rothbart, 2007). Additionally, the ability to engage in the flexible and adaptive mode of attention called "attentional switching" is also consistent with this model (Mirsky, Anthony, Duncan, Ahearn, & Kellam, 1991). There are clear parallels between these different qualities of attention and the mindfulness practices that are specifically designed to help the individual place and hold the attention where he or she wants it, and to notice various mental experiences as they arise.

Attention has been described as situated action or patterns of behavioral control that are influenced by the individual's current context and history (Hayes & Shenk, 2004). Within mindfulness, attention can be defined as "a focusing of an awareness to highlight selected aspects of that reality" (Brown & Ryan, 2004, p. 243). Additionally, one goal of such attentional training is to discipline the naturally wandering mind (Kwee, 2011a). Mindfulness involves the self-regulation of many attentional processes in order to maintain choiceless awareness. This self-regulation of attention from moment to moment is comprised of selectively focused, sustained, and switching of attention. This also includes executive attention, in service of nonelaborative processing and nonattachment, thus allowing the individual to observe where the mind naturally wanders without elaborating on these wanderings and instead letting go and redirecting attention back toward present moment awareness (Hayes & Feldman, 2004).

Both psychologists and Buddhist scholars would agree that intentional, selective, and sustained attention to particular stimuli requires the ability to monitor awareness and the focus of attention, detecting and not engaging in distraction, and redirecting and engaging attention to the intended stimulus (Lutz, Slagter, Dunne, & Davidson, 2008; Lutz et al. 2009). Sustained attention involves the ability to maintain vigilance over a single point of awareness for a substantial period of time. Selective attention is "the capacity for or process of reacting to certain stimuli selectively when several occur simultaneously" (*Oxford Dictionary*, 1989). Switching allows for the redirection of attention back to the object of focus or awareness. A small but methodologically diverse body of research supports a proposed relationship between mindfulness and the capacity for sustained attention, selective attention, and attentional switching (Chambers et al., 2008; Fulton & Seigel, 2005; Jha, Krompinger, & Baime, 2007; Josefsson & Broberg, 2010; Pagnoni & Cekic, 2007; Valentine & Sweet, 1999). These studies approached mindfulness from a number of different perspectives, variously examining experienced meditators, mindfulness-based meditation interventions such as MBSR, and trait or dispositional mindfulness.

In general, results from these studies reveal improvements in attention processes over the course of one's experience and time spent with mindfulness meditation and training. For example, one study conducted by Jha and colleagues (2007) examined three groups: a group of experienced meditators before and after an intensive 1-month retreat, a group of novice meditators before and after an 8-week MBSR training course, and a control group measured 8 weeks apart. In this study, selective attention was demonstrated as superior in both the experienced meditators and those in the MBSR group as compared to controls. However, sustained attention enhancement was more significant in the group of nonexperienced MBSR participants compared to the experienced meditators after the 1-month intensive retreat and control groups. No significant differences were observed between novice MBSR participants and novice control group individuals on tasks involving sustained attention (Jha et al., 2007). These results seem to indicate that enhancement of selective attention is more notable in individuals who are just beginning mindfulness training or practice, versus those who are more expert and possibly advanced in terms of maintaining this mindful attention and awareness, indicating a possible ceiling effect occurring as individuals practice over time. Individuals who have longer-term, more advanced experience with mindfulness meditation tend to perform better on tasks of sustained attention when compared with matched controls (Pagnoni & Cekic, 2007). Furthermore, sustained and selective attention are also positively correlated with self-reported levels of dispositional mindfulness (Moore & Malinowski, 2009).

Similarly, research also reveals enhanced attention-switching abilities in more advanced mindfulness practitioners (Chiesa, Calati, & Serretti, 2011). Long-term, experienced meditators have demonstrated the ability to provide a greater number of different perspectives in response to ambiguous stimuli and to identify their initial perception more rapidly than individuals with no meditation experience (Hodgin & Adair, 2010). However, other studies have failed to show significant differences between control groups and individuals who have completed a shorter-term mindfulness training or practice (Anderson, Lau, Segal, & Bishop, 2007; Chambers, Lo, & Allen, 2008; Heeren, Van Broeck, & Philippot, 2009). With regard to research on attentional switching, executive attention, and mindfulness research, some studies have revealed positive correlations between mindfulness training experience and higher Stroop scores (Chan & Woollacott, 2007; Moore & Malinowski, 2009; Van den Hurk et al., 2010). Switching helps the individual remain present-centered and prevents him or her from being influenced by history or context, or by being hijacked by habitual or dysfunctional thought processes and responses (Bishop, 2002; Hayes & Shenk, 2004).

These various aspects of attention are important in helping individuals to interface adaptively with often rapidly shifting aspects of their internal and external realities. Selective and sustained attention provide the capacity to attend to all of the available stimuli in a given moment and the utilization of switching allows the attentional process to continue and flow with the ever-changing present moment. All of these attentional processes are essential elements in the cultivation of mindfulness and mind training in Buddhist psychology.

The utilization of switching allows for the inhibition of elaborative processing, which can also be referred to as *bare attention* or attending "to the bare facts of perception without reacting to them by deed, speech or mental comment" (Nyanaponika Thera, 1962, p. 3). Bare attention offers raw, unrefined experience of the present moment (Nyanaponika Thera, 1962). It has been suggested that this type of noninvolvement with stimuli is most likely related to the unattached nature of mindful awareness, free from conceptualizations, evaluations, or emotional classifications that skew "pure" or "lucid" contact with the present moment (Das, 1997). With bare attention, an individual resists making judgments, considering implications, or interpreting or acting on these experiences (Bishop, 2002). Without judgment, individuals have the ability to see things as they are and nothing more (Germer, 2005a). This type of processing allows mindfulness practice to help individuals resist engaging in ruminative or depressogenic thought patterns (Chambers et al., 2008; Ramel, Goldin, Carmona, & McQuaid, 2004; Teasdale et al., 1995). It has been suggested that individuals who practice mindfulness may gain improved cognitive inhibition, especially with regards to stimulus selection, and may free up cognitive resources by not engaging in elaborative processes (Bishop et al., 2004).

Buddhist psychology traditions involve numerous exercises and meditation training approaches that aim to develop the mindfulness quality of bare attention. In the Western world, perhaps one of the most well known of these approaches involves Zen meditation. Maintaining a beginner's mind, or *shoshin* in Japanese, is an essential part of many Buddhist and Zen traditions (Suzuki, 1970). The qualities of a beginner's mind include openness, receptiveness, and readiness to learn (Goodman, 2005). One might also assert that these are also desirable qualities in a therapist (or a patient for that matter). In fact, beginner's mind is similar to the curious, empirical approach that is often used in various forms of CBT techniques for both therapist (e.g., Socratic questioning) and patient. The goal is to maintain a consistent fresh perspective or "original mind" (Suzuki, 1970, p. 21). Mindfulness utilizes the perspective of a beginner's mind, which involves addressing awareness of various objects, sensations, thoughts, or feelings as they arise as if for the first time, each time they arise. In beginner's mind, there are no self-centered thoughts to cloud and limit perception, which allows one to see things as they really are and begin to learn the true nature of things (Suzuki, 1970). Remaining in a beginner or novice mode of perception provides freedom from preconceived, conditioned notions and beliefs that might block or skew experience (Bishop et al., 2004). Just as in CBT, where certain core beliefs or dysfunctional schemas distort and conceptualize our world based on prior events, learning, and other non-present-centered influences, beginner's mind also aims to unglue an individual from his or her expectations, and to look at what really is, right now. Thus, continuing to uphold this fresh, open perspective and refraining from elaborating on present experience can help individuals prevent themselves from absorption in categorical and evaluative thinking that often disrupts the experience of the present moment and filters the way in which we view ourselves and our world (Bishop et al., 2004; Hayes & Shenk, 2004).

Beginner's mind and the practice of mindfulness has been said to interfere with the process of habituation. Early research with four experienced Zen masters revealed EEG patterns that demonstrated a lack of habituation to a repeated clicking sound compared to nonmeditators, who showed typical patterns of habituation (Kasamatsu & Hirai, 1973). While this study's findings have yet to be replicated, the replication attempt by Becker and Shapiro (1981) used different groupings of meditators and controls, different sound characteristics and method of delivery, and the controls were not matched for age. So while more research is clearly needed before definitive statements can be made in regard to habituation and mindfulness, if meditation and mindfulness training created more "space between impulse and reaction," then this may in fact be a useful tool in slowing down automatic, habitual processes such as distorted thinking patterns. Mindfulness strips away distortion and reminds us that the only reality that exists is right now, providing more accurate directly sourced information from the current context.

The fourth and final foundation of mindfulness is *Dhammas*, which can be translated as mental contents or phenomena, or "mental projections." This can be considered mindfulness of the mind, the application of mindful awareness to one's own mental activities, which has obvious implications for effectively working with emotional difficulties. This practice rests in the notion of interdependence in perception, in that nothing exists separately from the being who perceives it. Research has associated mindfulness with reductions in avoidance behaviors, thought suppression, and other dysfunctional processes associated with psychological disorders. For example, research has found that an 8-week mindfulness-based intervention is effective in significantly reducing anxiety and depressive symptoms in patients with generalized anxiety and panic disorders (Kabat-Zinn et al., 1992). These results were retained at 3-year follow-up (Miller, Fletcher, & Kabat-Zinn, 1995). Additionally, mindfulness practice has been associated with decreases in dysfunctional cognitions such as rumination and worry (Bishop et al., 2004; Hayes & Feldman, 2004; Roemer & Orsillo, 2002; Teasdale et al., 1995, 2000), which can also be viewed as a form of avoidance (Borkovec & Roemer, 1995; Roemer & Orsillo, 2002). Rumination can be considered an opposite process in comparison to mindfulness. This kind of restrictive thinking can exacerbate negative thoughts and emotions and pull an individual out of the reality of the present moment, submerging him or her in perseverative thought patterns involving the past, fantasy, or the future (Bishop et al., 2004; Brown & Ryan, 2003; Nolen-Hoekensema, 2000). Mindfulness allows for a decrease in goal-based modes of processing such as rumination and worry, and allows individuals to utilize a contrary mode of processing that is not goal-based (Teasdale, Segal, & Williams, 2003). This new perspective can change the experience of emotions, so that one's feelings or emotions do not unduly influence one's understanding and reasoning.

HEALTHY THOUGHT AND UNDERSTANDING

Traditional *Right View* or *Right Understanding* involves insight into and knowledge of the theory, processes, and overall phenomenology proposed by Buddhist psychology. At the core of this knowledge is an understanding of the two truths, Buddhist psychology views of reality, and the nature of suffering, including its causes and its alleviation. More specifically, it is a deep understanding that comes with experiential learning and examination of the four immeasurables, the seven factors of the awakened mind, the Four Noble Truths, and the Eightfold Path. Buddhist psychology posits that these realizations create the necessary conditions for nonattachment or nonclinging to unpleasant and pleasant experiences, which leads to liberation from suffering and the freedom to choose how one wants to act in the world (Olendzki, 2010).

Healthy Understanding and the Two-Truth Theory

The Two-Truth Theory reflects the Buddhist view of the layers of truth (Dalai Lama, 1991). The first truth is an empirical, phenomenal, and relativistic perspective on the things we perceive that enter our conscious awareness. The second truth concerns the deeper, fundamental, or ultimate nature of reality: emptiness (*Sunyata*). As we have discussed, Buddhist psychology understands that the our reality functions in terms of interdependence and impermanence, a constantly changing whole made up of constantly changing parts, producing an illusion of a fixed reality. The concept of "interdependent origination" is a fundamental view in Buddhism and emphasizes causation in the determination of existence (Dalai Lama, 1991).

Buddhism identifies the two central forms of causation as internal and external. External forms of causation can be seen as public events or objects, and examples of internal causes are thoughts, feelings, or private events (Dalai Lama, 1991). These causes are directly related to our experiences of suffering and those conditions that impact our behavior. Hence, Buddhist psychology hypothesizes a transactional and intricate relationship between internal and external causes, which reflects an ongoing, interactive system of causes and conditions that function to produce an individual's experience of reality. In the Buddhist endeavor to understand the mind, it is critical to not focus solely on the internal workings of the mind—its mental and cognitive events— but to also understand their relationship with the external world and a given context, or the relationships between "mind and matter" (Dalai Lama, 1991, p. 16). In a sense, every practitioner of the *dharma* is his or her own scientist, on an empirical journey. Much like a behaviorist scientist-practitioner, the Buddhist practitioner is less concerned with finding out the "absolute truth" in terms of the ontological nature of reality, and is more concerned with successful working in terms of freedom from suffering. Within Buddhist psychology seldom is one aspect or component of the Eightfold Path applied in isolation and instead each supports one another and are often related to ethics, values, and "workability."

Healthy Thinking

The Buddhist psychology approach to *Healthy Thought* is rather nuanced, in that it ultimately involves mindful nonattachment from the contents of thought (particularly in the case of unhelpful thoughts that fuel problematic affective responses), combined with the purposeful cultivation of helpful ways of thinking, in the recognition that, in fact, thoughts and imagery can indeed serve as causes and conditions that can positively impact our emotional well-being. Approaching our thinking in a way that is consistent with practicing the Middle Path intervention not only includes increased perception, it also promotes additional cognitive change through both alterations in thought patterns and differences in the way one looks at or feels about his or her cognitions (Baer, 2003; Kabat-Zinn, 1990, 2003; Teasdale, 1999). Buddhist psychology provides insight into the true nature of cognitions and affect, viewing them as transient mental events that are not a direct reflection of reality or of the self (Bishop et al., 2004). Mindfulness may also contribute to cognitive complexity by increasing the generation of distinct and integrated understanding of cognitions and affect (Bishop et al., 2004). This can involve a new understanding of thoughts, feelings, and actions and their relationships with one another. Mindfulness is positively correlated with psychological mindedness, which is defined as the ability to reflect on the relationship between thoughts, emotions, and actions (Beitel, Ferrer, & Cerero, 2005; Bishop et al., 2004).

As mentioned above, another aspect of *Healthy Thought* in Buddhist psychology is the purposeful cultivation of healthy patterns of thinking such as the cultivation of compassionate thinking and imagery. Kelly, Zuroff, and Shapira (2009) investigated the effects of imagery-guided self-help techniques for either self-soothing or resisting self-attacks in people with severe acne and related distress. The self-soothing condition, derived from compassion-focused imagery, included daily practice in imagining a source of compassion and repeating nurturing self-statements. Individuals in the attack-resisting condition were trained to generate a strong and resilient image and to repeat statements meant to retaliate against their inner critic such as "I have the inner strength to fight my distress and your role in creating it" (Kelly et al., 2009, pp. 306–307). Results showed that self-soothing thoughts decreased shame and skin complaints, but not depression; and attack-resisting thoughts lowered all three.

This outcome may be related to preliminary findings that people with depression and anxiety perceive self-compassion to be a very difficult standpoint to adopt, especially in the context of their disorders (Pauley & McPherson, 2010). It could also be understood in light of a finding that, compared to controls, depressed individuals show a preference for self-punishment, which rapidly reduces their levels of autonomic tension (Forrest & Hokanson, 1975); this evidence indicates that self-punishment may actually have some soothing qualities for people with depression (e.g., familiarity), and might explain why it is such a difficult habit to change.

Research examining compassion interventions that target the cognitive process highlights cognitive reframing as an important mechanism of action. By helping people become more mindful, empathic, and aware that suffering and imperfection are part of the human condition, compassion and self-compassion training promote more adaptive cognitive schemas around experiences of suffering and struggle. In facilitating a shift from a perspective that views one's struggles and suffering as indicative of fundamental flaws in one's nature to a position in which these difficult experiences are seen as common elements that bind all human beings together, one can powerfully alter both one's relationship to the suffering as well as to the intra- and interpersonal meaning carried by the suffering.

A number of researchers have also begun to examine the effects of compassion interventions for people with psychosis. Though small-scale and uncontrolled, the interventions featured in these pilot studies have yielded encouraging effects. Mayhew and Gilbert (2008) found that group CFT had the effects of decreasing participants' levels of depression, anxiety, paranoia, obsessive–compulsive tendencies, psychoticism, and interpersonal sensitivity. Perhaps most impressively, this intervention influenced the quality of participants' auditory hallucinations, which became less malevolent and persecuting and more reassuring. Another intervention modeled on CFT was conducted in a maximum-security hospital for individuals with psychosis and violent/criminal propensities (Laithwaite et al., 2009); results showed significant changes in levels of depression and self-esteem, and moderate decreases in feelings of inferiority to others and in general psychopathology. Relatedly, LKM has been associated with decreases in negative symptoms, especially anhedonia, and increased frequency of positive emotions in patients with psychosis (Johnson et al., 2009).

LIMITATIONS AND FUTURE DIRECTIONS

The research we have examined here includes a number of significant and novel findings. However, there is much work yet to be done to expand the existing literature base and to address limitations present in many of the studies in this area. Many studies utilized small samples, did not randomize to active and control conditions, and/or focused solely on immediate benefits. Often the measures at the disposal of researchers in this area are limited to self-report questionnaires. Other critiques of Buddhist psychology-related research highlight a number of methodological issues and challenges. For example, in a literature review, many meditation interventions for anxiety treatment do not meet the required methodological inclusion criteria (Krisanaprakornkit, Krisanaprakornkit, Piyavhatkul, & Laopaiboon, 2005).

There are challenges in teaching mindfulness, and the effectiveness of mindfulness training procedures still requires more research (Dimidjian & Linehan, 2003; Kabat-Zinn, 2003). Some of these programs are more demanding than others in that some programs require strict adherence to practice schedules or recording requirements (Kabat-Zinn, 1990), sometimes leading to high attrition rates (Baer, 2003). Despite these and other methodological difficulties, this research shows promise: mindfulness-based interventions seem to be efficacious and may be helpful in the treatment of a variety of disorders and possibly improve functioning research. Finally, while a good bit of research has been conducted on mindfulness in recent decades, considerably more study needs to be conducted to explore the theory and practice of other aspects of Buddhist psychology that have found their way into the therapy room, such as the cultivation of compassion and loving-kindness, as well as Buddhist psychology-inspired imagery exercises such as those seen in compassionate mind training. All in all, it is probably fair to say that the empirical investigation of Buddhist psychology is still in its infancy, and it is our hope that this book might inspire further interest and research in these areas.

The Question of Enlightenment
and Case Formulation

> If you have knowledge, let others light their candles
> in it.
>
> —MARGARET FULLER

THE QUESTION OF ENLIGHTENMENT FOR CBT

In the West we understand and codify Buddhism as a form of religion and CBT as a form of applied science. As a result, those of us who have consciously adopted a scientific worldview are rightly careful before adopting therapeutic methods that have emerged from religious traditions—and thus rightly cautious as we encounter Buddhist psychology. However, Buddhism diverges from Western ideas about what a religion constitutes in many ways. Buddhism is not a theistic system of philosophy, and it makes no assertions about whether there is a God or gods. Additionally, much of what occurs in a typical CBT session is likely as informed by moment-by-moment apprehension of the emotions in a holistic, nonspecific fashion as it is by hard science. In truth, neither system is entirely scientific, nor entirely based in speculation. At its core, Buddhism does not involve supernatural or spiritual assumptions (Kwee et al., 2006). Of course, in its various forms over the centuries, Buddhism has adopted a variety of mythopoetic and culturally situated ideas and symbols, such as images of radiant *Bodhisattvas* or a belief in reincarnation. However, the Buddha himself famously refused to say whether he believed there were divine powers or life after death, encouraging his disciples to follow their own lines of inquiry and come to their own conclusions (Rahula, 1959/1974). Despite this abandonment of a theistic approach by Buddhism, and the widespread adoption of Buddhist practices by Western psychologists, some ideas from Buddhism remain difficult to touch from a scientific worldview. Notably, the central aim of all of Buddhist philosophy and practice, the process of achieving enlightenment, is one such idea that is rarely discussed in CBT circles, let alone the broader scientific community.

Indeed, when we discuss the concept of achieving enlightenment in terms of CBT, we find ourselves in territory that appears outside of the domain of clinical psychology, and working with ideas that may be better relegated to the domain of spirituality or religion. However, just a short while ago this is exactly what we might have said about the entire range of meditation principles that are now central to neuroscience and psychology.

It is important, of course, to temper any enthusiasm to explore the application of prescientific concepts with a rigorous application of our scientific principles. However, the ideal of an enlightened mind is central to Buddhist psychology, and understanding this ideal can allow us to approach the integration of Buddhist psychology and CBT with greater wisdom and more skillful means. Furthermore, if we approach the scholarship, teachings, and intellectual efforts of literally millions of people within the Buddhist tradition with too narrow a Western lens, aren't we bringing a set of repertoire-narrowing, and perhaps even culturally prejudiced, assumptions to our analyses? If we allow ourselves to impart legitimacy to a brain scan and self-report assessment of one meditator who has done an 8-week mindfulness course *studied by a major North American university*, but ignore centuries of scholarship, knowledge development, and subjective empirical inquiry *engaged in by thousands of experts in Asian monasteries*, what sort of a filter are we using in our scientific integration of the body of global human knowledge? If we selectively focus our analysis on a few elements of Buddhist psychology, such as mindfulness and acceptance, simply because they have already been comodified, branded, and legitimized by mainstream academia, aren't we being more guided by our reified assumptions about social structures than by a focus on comprehensive knowledge development? The idea of enlightenment is at the core of Buddhist psychology, and the metaphor of awakening is central to enlightenment. Engaging with these ideas from a scientifically grounded perspective can provide a deeper understanding of Buddhist psychology for the CBT practitioner, and may provide a new lens for case formulation and treatment development.

LIGHT, ENLIGHTENMENT, AND AWAKENING

The metaphor of light in spiritual and philosophical traditions carries a great many associations and stimulus functions for us, and has been used across the world since the beginning of social history. Islam, Taoism, Christianity, Hinduism, Judaism, and even the "secular enlightenment" of Western empiricism have all used the metaphor of light to describe an increase in a human's knowledge, appreciation, wisdom, and direct experience of the nature of reality. Interestingly, we now know that the activity of our networked brain and central nervous system involves electrochemical synaptic transmission that involves energy exchanges similar to that of light, which comprises electrical and magnetic activity. Furthermore, light can stimulate our mental activity and increase our alertness, cognitive performance, wakefulness, and positive affect (Austin, 1999; Vanderwalle et al., 2013). Recent research has demonstrated that exposure to blue light can even stimulate cognitive activity and enhance alertness in visually blind individuals (Vanderwalle et al., 2013). Even with complete lack of sight, some human beings are sensitive to the presence of light, and this sensitivity influences the default mode network of the brain so that it remains alert and attentive to activity in the outside world and to imaginal experience.

Indeed, light regulates our sleep, wakes us from dreams, and modulates the degree to which we respond to mental stimuli as if they were things in the outside world. In terms of the rhythm of our biological functioning, we have evolved to rest and descend into sleep when light is absent. During this sleep, our mental experiences present themselves to our nonconscious awareness in the form of dreams, which present themselves as entirely literal. Indeed, if it were not for our endogenously created muscle paralysis during sleep, it is hypothesized that stimuli in dream states would influence us to move our bodies in the real world. We have similarly evolved to awaken when the presence of light in the world is sensed biologically, awakening electrical processes that fuel and enable our neural network to form conscious experience of the outside world. In this way, light triggers us to awaken, and to respond to our environment more adaptively, and treat our thoughts, images, and emotions as mental events rather than as things in the world. Hence, light, awakening, and functioning adaptively with an accurate perception of the actuality of our situation are intimately interdependent.

Rather than a supernatural and cosmic divine light that imparts some sort of spiritual power, the enlightenment we are referring to in Buddhist psychology suggests the process of waking up, as is suggested by the original Sanskrit term for enlightenment, *Bodhi*, and the Japanese term *Satori*, which mean "awakened." Similarly, an alternative Japanese term for sudden enlightenment, *Kensho*, means "seeing one's true nature" (Austin, 1999). The *Shamballa Dictionary of Buddhism and Zen* defines enlightenment as follows: "A person awakens to a newness of emptiness, which he himself is—even as the entire universe is emptiness—and which alone enables him to comprehend the true nature of things" (Shamballa, 1991, p. 65).

According to this definition, the term "awakening mind" is preferable to "enlightenment." When we examine the aims of Buddhist practice, the metaphor of waking up is a closer approximation of the phenomenon described than the idea of enlightenment. This phenomenon, and the reality of directly experiencing a state of awakening, however fleeting or enduring, is not an abstraction or cosmic transformation in Buddhism, but stands for an attainable human capacity to develop our faculties of experiencing to a point where we are able more accurately to contact the experience of being, in a maximally adaptive manner that involves a dissolution of the experience of individual suffering.

When "emptiness" is referred to in Buddhist psychology, it is important to remember that we are not speaking of vacuity or nihilism. Emptiness (*Shunyata*) is understood in two primary schools of thought in Buddhism (Thurman, 1997). The first approach, known as the "mind only" (*yogachara*) understanding of emptiness, recognizes that all that we formulate and represent in our conscious awareness is, literally, the product and process of mental activity alone. In this way, everything that is perceived is empty of existence separate from the act of perception. In the second understanding of emptiness, known as the "middle" (*Madhyamika*) school, emptiness is understood as representing the degree to which every aspect of reality is intimately interwoven with a myriad of conditions. This school of thought observes that if we are to break down the constituents of any phenomenon to the most basic units of measurement, we will ultimately reduce the observable phenomena into a point where distinctions and separateness become irrelevant or impossible to logically sustain. This idea can be illustrated by currently popular scientific concepts such as quantum physics or neural network theory. For example, the solidity of observable physical elements gradually seems less solid when we look at things at the quantum level, where the distinction between wave and particle becomes less defined. In such a paradigm, all phenomena can even be viewed as involving vibrating "strings" of nonlocal, interacting probabilities of energetic activity. In another example, the solidity of our sense of self or even the action of a unitary brain or mind is described as emerging from patterns of spreading activation of network nodes in neural network activity. When we look for separateness and permanence in our analysis of the observable world, we are ultimately led to the ongoing interdependent origination of elements that have no identity without existing in impermanent relation to one another. Furthermore, all of this only comes into being through the perspective of an observer. "Emptiness" in this sense represents the ultimate lack of separateness and lack of inherent existence for all things.

The extension of the Madhyamika philosophy suggests that phenomena are so interrelated and things so connected to one another that distinctions and illusions of separateness all arise through the illusion of a self and self–other relationships inherent in mental functioning. Approaching an awakening mind, then, represents a process of gradually and directly coming into experiential knowledge of the nature of reality, in the present moment, beyond representational mediation of experience through verbal processing or propositional knowledge structures. To be fully here and now, beyond concepts of self in relation to other, here in relation to there, now in relation to then, and even beyond having these concepts as referents, approaches the phenomenon of the awakening mind described in Buddhist psychology.

THE AWAKENING MIND EXPRESSED IN OUR BRAINS AND BEHAVIOR

Reflecting upon mental activity as an expression of the actions of the brain, Richard Davidson has described Buddhist practices employed in pursuit of awakening as "a form of mental training that involves the voluntary alteration of patterns of neural activity, and can have effects on peripheral biology through these mechanisms" (Davidson, 2011, p. 47). From a certain point of view, any form of mental training will alter patterns of neural activity. However, as we have surveyed the research on Buddhist meditation, we have concluded that Buddhist psychology involves training the orientation of our attention in purposeful and deliberate ways, which can give rise to new, unpredictable patterns of neural behavior that indirectly bring about greater mental and physical health. These changes are not limited to changes in cognitive content, or even to our attitudes and ideas about this cognitive content. Throughout this text, we have observed how research increasingly demonstrates that training in Buddhist meditation can result in positive, functional changes in immune and endocrine systems, as well as neural systems involved in anxiety, secure attachment, and mood. Among many other scientists and practitioners, Davidson posits that levels of positive affect, dimensions of attention, and degrees of compassion can be increased through the training of specific mental skills. Each of these skills is an element of the awakening mind. We will experience individual differences in our capacity for emotion regulation, cognitive styles, and various psychological capacities, based on the causal chains that are involved in our genetic inheritance and social learning histories. However, beyond how we emerge in the world, and how we are shaped by our learning history, we have the capacity to cultivate certain capacities that can contribute to our liberation from suffering and to our waking up in the present moment.

AWAKENING WISDOM, EMOTIONS, AND RATIONALITY

As we have seen, cognitive and behavioral therapies share an obvious common ground with training to wake up from illusory views of reality. Beyond a similarity of technique, it is possible that both Western and Eastern traditions of emotional healing may be pointing to a similar "true north" of realized, adaptive human potential. At its core, the central premise of all of the generations and variations of CBT involves the ability to train the mind in new perspectives and new ways of viewing reality. Whether cognitive change is pursued as an aim in itself, or whether new ways of thinking are construed as a part of a contextual strategy for broadening the behavioral repertoire of an individual, the various forms of CBT aim to offer new ways of knowing and acting that diminish our suffering and bring us into more adaptive mental functioning. Despite the reference to cognition and behavior in the name "cognitive-behavioral therapy," working with the emotions, particularly the presence of emotional pain, is a key focus of most interventions.

Emotions have great influence on our motivation, physical health, and behavior, and arise in an interdependent relationship with our cognitions and verbal processes. The experience of emotions, as expressed in the behavior of the human brain, involves many different interconnected structures that have a range of functions, and that demonstrate the activity of a distributed processing system. For example, the prefrontal cortex, which is involved in our thinking, planning, and derived relational responding, also is involved in the regulation of emotional responding, through its action upon the amygdala, insula, and ventral striatum. Notably, there is a bidirectional relationship between these structures and other systems in the body, such as the autonomic nervous system and the immune system. This makes sense when we realize that there is a bidirectionality to our experience of emotions in the body, and our cognitions and verbal behavior about our emotions. According to Davidson, "When we change the brain, we inevitably influence the body . . . when the body changes, it in turn influences the brain" (Davidson, 2011). The concepts of interdependent origination and bidirectional relational responding are physically mirrored, in a sense, in the behavior of the physical systems of a human being, as an embodied cognitive presence.

As we experience the balance of cognition, physical sensation, and emotional experience, we encounter wisdom. Clearly, the sort of holistic knowing that is described in an awakened state involves the highest order of wisdom. In common use, the term "wisdom" refers to our ability to make decisions, rely upon our own judgment, and implies the coming together of a variety of mental capacities. These capacities suggest an ability to appreciate reality on its own terms, including discernment, insight, and the ability to view things rationally (Seigel & Germer, 2013). However, the rationality that is enacted with a wise mind is far more than the cold logic that many might associate with being "rational." Rational wisdom involves a form of viewing the world that relates to the original definition of *ratio*, involved in being rational, involving an ability to view experiences and changes in the environment in proportion to one another.

Such wisdom is discussed as a desirable state of mind in the heavily Buddhist influenced DBT (Linehan, 1993a). DBT describes a balanced blend of emotional processing and intellectual processing as a "wise mind" perspective. This wise mind allows an individual to synthesize his or her motivational and emotional processing with his or her logical faculties, to make sound judgments, and to live life in an adaptive and meaningful way. Learning to integrate the information inherent in our emotional responding with our rational minds results in a wisdom that points in the direction of liberation from suffering, nonetheless. Given the popularity and effectiveness of DBT in treating challenging problems in emotion regulation, it is safe to assume that thousands of Westerners are learning to pursue the wisdom of the awakening mind as you are reading these words, without realizing that the alleviation of their suffering has its seeds in the discoveries of Buddhist practitioners or giving a second thought to a concept of enlightenment. The concept of "enlightenment" in such cases is not important as a thing in itself, and, in Buddhist psychology terms, is never important beyond its impermanent nature as a signifier for our waking up.

Some perspectives on wisdom suggest that it represents a triumph of the cognitive faculties over our emotional motivations, in a quintessence of top-down processing (Seigel & Germer, 2013). In this conceptualization of wisdom, the higher cortical functioning involved in our executive functions and conceptual schemas exerts a great degree of influence and perhaps control over our emotions and conditioned responses. However compelling this view of wisdom may be, it is difficult to establish evidence to support a hard cognitive meditation perspective on the wisdom of the awakened mind as pointed to by a Buddhist understanding.

As one case of awakening wisdom, let's look at the balanced neural activity present in accessing mindfulness and compassion. In the case of mindfulness and compassion, both top-down and bottom-up processes are necessary to bring our old brain motivations into coordinated action with our new brain capabilities. Emotional-processing centers located deep in the brain (which have an ancient evolutionary history and are involved in human attachment emotions) are necessary to stimulate the parasympathetic nervous system and the vasovagal complex, facilitating stillness, centering, and a sense of compassionate safeness (Porges, 1995). From such a place, our flexible perspective-taking, mentalization, and meta-awareness abilities may all be activated, allowing us to experience mindfulness and one-pointed concentration. Accordingly, rather than awakening involving a rarefied and precise form of top-down mental organization, the emergence of wisdom actually involves neural and behavioral integration of the highest order, where the myriad of streams of information that may inform our behavior are balanced, and we may come that much closer to experiencing the world just as it is. In this way, wisdom involves us bringing all of ourselves, all of the aggregate and interrelated elements of our being, to bear upon our moment-by-moment experience, allowing us to "wake up" to the nature of "suchness," which is precisely what Buddhist psychology has suggested is involved in the experience of enlightenment, realization, or awakening. So, the process of waking up suggests, in many ways, the synthesis of a range of these interdependent elements of human mental functioning. Implicit and explicit memories and processing are involved when we base our worldview and actions upon our wise mind. Our emotional memories are involved, as are our valued aims, when we seek to wake up, and live our lives fully and meaningfully.

The wisdom of the awakening mind, which is traditionally described as the perfection of transcendent wisdom (*prajna paramita*), can emerge through training in mindfulness, acceptance, compassion, and concentration, and go beyond living lives of contentment that are identified with our self story. Furthermore, such wisdom goes beyond even contentedly abiding in a mindful experience of the present moment from the perspective of the observing self. According to Buddhist psychology, deeper levels of meditation and mental training can effect an experience of self, wherein the mental construction of self and other, experiencer and experienced, begin to wholly dissolve. In Buddhist psychology terms, this experience mirrors a direct understanding, and perhaps embodiment of the essential emptiness, and lack of inherent existence of all things, *shunyata*. As we have discussed *shunyata*, the metaphor of emptiness, does not reflect an infinite barrenness or hollow universe as much as it is meant to point to the unboundaried and perhaps boundless contour of an undivided universe, a domain of infinite potential that literally is beyond what a human intelligence would define as space and time. This understanding of things as they are involves an inherent compassion that perhaps arises in a nonverbally mediated way, which is to say that it is not representative and symbolic but an emergent emotional knowing, inexpressible, undivided, and infinitely in expression of an extended present moment. Just as Taoists would proclaim that "the Tao that can be told is not the eternal Tao," there is a wisdom in the experience of emptiness that goes beyond our capacity to derive relations, carve up reality, or form verbal expressions of the absolute. This sort of knowing is viewed as the source of *prajna paramita.*

Just as we are able to use our computers and our mobile phones with a graphic user interface, rather than reading the millions of lines of binary code or deciphering the patterns of countless electric circuits that go into reading a book on a tablet computer, we do not approach *prajna paramita* by abandoning our mental faculties or by disengaging from reality. As we noted in the discussion of the "two truth" theory, our appreciation of absolute truth is approached through relative truth. We engage with and communicate the way to approach awakening wisdom through our capacity for language, cognition, and emotional comprehension. Of course, the moment that we begin to relate, frame, or conceptualize experience in human terms, then cognition and our learning histories will influence the experience and its communication. However, through training in meditative awareness, Buddhist psychology suggests that we can cultivate and draw upon our own inherently enlightened nature to increase our capacity to live in the world awake, aware and sensitive to the suffering that we encounter. Buddhist psychology suggests that our experience of the altruistic aspiration to alleviate the suffering of all beings—innate enlightened mind of *bodhicitta*—is *the* key to the process of gradually awakening and establishing an enlightened mind. As this is the path to the alleviation of suffering, the mental training involved becomes very important within Buddhist traditions. Regardless of whether the concept of awakening appears important to the CBT practitioner, the mental experience that it points to, and the techniques of mental training that is has inspired, may be highly useful.

Awakening and Psychological Flexibility

When we begin to approach the concept of the awakening mind in terms of CBT interventions, we are talking about a personal transformation that is a full realization and further extension of the concepts of psychological flexibility, mindfulness, and compassion. The values, behaviors, sense of self, and attentional stance that are involved in the awakened state of mind, however, are not of a personal nature, but of an experientially transpersonal nature. The perspective that is taken is wholly dis-identified, and the valued directions that are pursued are entirely related to liberation from attachment and defusion from the very mental constructs that establish the parameters of a substantial reality as we understand it. Willingness to experience pain—complete willingness to endure the pain of absence and the pain of presence—is a large constituent of this maximally adaptive variation upon the theme of psychological flexibility. Pain itself experienced from the perspective of such a disidentified state ceases to be pain in the sense that we know pain. Time and space are experienced from behind and above the verbal relations that bring these concepts into being. From the liberated and enlightened perspective, they cease to exist in any context of literality at all. From the reported neurophenomenology of advanced meditators, the experience of the awakening mind has the quality of spaciousness, interiority, and luminosity. Historically, in Buddhist psychology, this is the "Clear Light" (*prabhasvara*) that the concept of enlightenment points to. These metaphors and words signify a human potential for freedom and for calm, in the presence of nearly any circumstance. This is not an ideal to be striven for, nor an end to be gained, but a reality of the ground of being that is supremely rational. The Socratic questioning that is involved in traditional cognitive therapy can be seen as a gentle approach to this ultimate awareness. The father of such rationality, Socrates, was an Orphic mystic, who very likely practiced a form of mindfulness that guided his method, so this makes a great deal of sense. The paths of human wisdom from East to West and West to East represent a flow of human behavioral and social evolution, and have been this way for far longer than we often appreciate.

THE SEVEN FACTORS OF THE AWAKENING MIND

Over the course of the last 2,600 years or so, Buddhist scholars have not simply elaborated their philosophical claims and left the community to struggle on their own. Rather, the tradition of the *Dharma* has consistently elaborated upon methods of engaged practice, in the form of numerous meditative techniques, visualization practices, and ethical guidelines. Additionally, Buddhism has a long tradition of texts and scriptures that elaborate and explain the various dimensions of the psychological landscape present in a Buddhist model of mind. As Buddhist psychology has evolved, various concepts have shifted in their emphasis, and have been delineated in greater detail. Among the many teachings elaborating dimensions of human mental functioning, *The Seven*

Factors of Awakening represent the qualities or characteristics that lead to individual enlightenment, and they have been the subject of core Buddhist teachings and numerous commentaries since the beginning of Buddhism. Initially, Buddhist texts, such as the biographical compendium of teachings known as the *dhammapada*, discuss these factors as wholesome mental states that can be pursued through practicing the *dharma*, and which may contribute to our waking up (Cleary, 1991). Later texts, such as the seminal mental road map of Buddhist psychology, *The Abidharma* (Goleman, 1988), discuss the factors of awakening more as emergent properties that arise within and from the process of enlightenment itself.

As CBT practitioners, our focus lies much more on the unfolding processes that can lead to the cessation of suffering and development of wisdom and compassion than it does on observing the qualities of an awakened being. As such, we will look at these factors of enlightenment as processes that might present themselves as potential areas of personal growth for our clients, and more in tune with their original conceptualization. In terms of case formulation, these seven factors may be understood as positive psychological states and traits that we may target through training in mindfulness, acceptance, compassion, and the Middle Path intervention. As we witness these factors growing in our clients, and in ourselves, we may notice a gradual movement toward a broader perspective and a loosening of maladaptive patterns of avoidance and attachment. As has always been the case, Buddhist psychology is a path of individual empiricism, and it is our aim to provide these dimensions of awakening in order to refocus our attention from clinical deficits to the unfolding strengths that may arise in response to training the mind through Buddhist psychology and CBT.

Near the end of his life, the Buddha spoke about the discoveries he encountered on his life's path and practice. In a short and renowned talk, the Buddha discussed particular qualities of mind and practices, including the "Seven Factors of Awakening." The processes and characteristics of the mind and heart that are outlined below are said to create the conditions or contexts that allow for the ability to release ourselves from clinging to, fusion with, and, ultimately, to liberation from suffering. These factors and their various processes are cultivated as inner strengths, resiliencies that facilitate the process of acceptance and letting go. Drawing from the psychological flexibility model (Hayes, Strosahl, & Wilson, 1999), we might refer to these factors as facilitating defusion, flexible perspective taking, staying in contact with the present moment, and openness to experience. In this way, we can formulate the function of "letting go" or nonattachment as providing us with choices and a wider range of options in how we choose to live and be in the world. Buddhist psychology would suggest that as these factors lead to increasing release from the cycle of attachment, avoidance, and suffering, that an inherent enlightened mind, steeped in compassion and wisdom, will arise in the practitioner. This is a hypothesis that has yet to be scientifically supported; however, we would invite the reader to conduct his or her own study of personal introspection, and explore this path with their fellow travelers—colleagues and clients alike. Buddhist psychology suggests that it is helpful to bring awareness and attention to the presence of these seven factors, taking note when they become apparent in us, showing them care, and cultivating them further. Importantly, the Seven Factors of Awakening are meant to contribute to well-being and have inherently reinforcing and motivating qualities that help an individual move toward what is workable and liberating in his or her mind and life. The factors can be translated in a number of ways, and we have transliterated these concepts with an eye toward integration with cognitive and behavioral practice.

1. Mindfulness in awakening (*sati-sambojjhanga*).
2. Investigation in awakening (*dhamma-vicaya-sambojjhanga*).
3. Persistence in awakening (*viriya-sambojjhanga*).
4. Happiness in awakening (*pīti-sambojjhanga*).
5. Serenity in awakening (*passaddhi-sambojjhanga*).
6. Concentration in awakening (*samādhi-sambojjhanga*).
7. Equanimity in awakening (*upekkhā-sambojjhanga*).

The third-wave CBT practitioner can immediately notice familiar elements among this list. Factors related to the experience of compassion and affiliative emotional activation are major elements of the constituents of the enlightened mind, such as serenity, equanimity, and joyfulness. Furthermore, states of flexible and focused attention, such as concentration and mindfulness, are also immediately apparent in the seven factors as in currently emerging CBT methods. Interestingly, the Pali term *viriya*, which is described as the third factor of awakening, is sometimes translated as "energy," and it implies a kind of energetic persistence that can fuel ongoing engagement with challenges. As we know, both persistence and accessing available motivational energy in life are aspects of personal commitment and well-being that are pursued through third-wave CBT. Finally, investigation, discernment, and analytic wisdom also contribute to these factors of the awakening mind. The application of such rationality and curiosity are hallmarks of the first decades of CBT technique and development, while such forms of reasoning are also involved in the authorship of valued aims. If particular skills that are trained in various CBT traditions are hypothesized as key factors in the development of an awakened mind, perhaps the integration of CBT does, indeed, involve the opportunity for more than the importing of Buddhist meditation methods into existing CBT modalities. It appears that CBT itself has specific training methods that work upon the hypothesized active processes in Buddhist psychology, leading directly to the state of well-being that is the ultimate aim of Buddhist practice.

Factor 1: Mindfulness in Awakening (*Sati-sambojjhanga*)

When Jon Kabat-Zinn chose mindfulness (*sati*) as the dimension of Buddhist practice that would serve as the foundation for his method of applying meditation to help persons with chronic illness, he was making a sound and logical choice, in terms of the factors of the awakening mind. Leading Buddhist teachers of our era, such as Chogyam Trungpa or Thich Nhat Hanh, have described mindfulness as the foundation upon which the rest of development in the *dharma* rests. If cultivating flexible-focused attention to the present moment with acceptance is the first factor in the liberation of an individual from needless suffering, then it is logical that the first factor in the liberation of the community of Western psychological science would be an immersion in mindfulness. Mindfulness allows us to consciously step out of the domination of our internal representations, to slow our goal-directed "autopilot" pursuits for a moment, and to allow things to be as they are. With mindfulness, our thoughts are thoughts, our emotions are emotions, and our physical sensations are physical sensations. If even for a moment, we are free to take in the whole of the situation, just as we might look down upon a village from a hilltop in the morning, seeing the movement of the entire scene, from the flow of the clouds to the opening of doors and windows to a new day. We are a part of the scene as the observer, and this may even be our own hometown, but we are not controlled by the comings and goings of the street from this vantage point. Mindfulness brings other factors of awakening into possibility.

Factor 2: Investigation in Awakening (*Dhamma-vicaya-sambojjhanga*)

When we have brought conscious attention to the present moment, have shifted perspective, and have decentered from identification and fusion with the contents of our consciousness, we are freer to explore and investigate what has been arising in the mind, and how we may wish to respond to these experiences. The second factor of awakening involves investigation of phenomena, within and without (*dharma pravi-chaya*). Worries and ruminations may draw us into preoccupation with the past or anxiety about the future, but our mindful stance allows us to investigate these mental events with a curiosity and an even-handed wisdom. We may ask ourselves, "What is my mind telling me?" or "What is going through my mind right now?", and respond with kindness and movement toward what matters most to us. Our innate wisdom and flexible perspective taking emerges from feeling centered in our place in an interwoven and interdependent fabric of reality. Rather than being enslaved to our habitual response patterns, our mindful investigation means we may choose new internal and external behaviors that serve our aim of awakening, reciprocally reinforcing our momentum on the path. We may investigate the origin of physical sensations that relate to emotions, by localizing emotion-related physical tension. Furthermore, we may choose to label our emotions, and develop more keen and adaptive awareness of what emotional and motivational systems are working upon and through us in the present moment. All of these elements of investigation are familiar to the CBT practitioner because the sequence of decentering, noticing automatic thoughts, observing physical responses to emotions, labeling our emotions, and choosing possible adaptive responses from the armamentarium of many CBT techniques, especially cognitive reframing, acceptance of anxiety, and enhancing emotional processing (Leahy, Tirch, & Napolitano, 2011). In Figure 10.1, we have provided a mindfulness- and acceptance-based thought record based on working with emotion regulation (Leahy et al., 2011). This "Emotionally Intelligent Thought Record" is an example of how CBT practitioners may choose to bring the factors of mindfulness and investigation into their work with persistent negative emotions and thoughts. According to Buddhist psychology, the factors of mindfulness and investigation may help our clients and ourselves to move into a place of greater wisdom and clear seeing. From such a space, we may find we are much better able to choose how we are in the world. What we do with this wisdom and perspective flows into (and from) the additional factors of the awakening mind.

The Emotionally Intelligent Thought Record: Awakening analytic reasoning.

Directions: Over the course of the next week, use this series of questions to help yourself practice a growing awareness of your thoughts, emotions, physical sensations, and possible responses. You can use this worksheet when you notice something affecting the way you are feeling, during times of stress, or even at times when you suddenly notice that your emotions have shifted in a negative direction. You can use this worksheet in "real time" to tune into what is going on in the present moment. Sometimes, though, this won't be possible. This is not a problem. You can still use this worksheet after some time has passed, by looking back upon your memories of an event, and asking yourself these questions as if things were happening in this moment. As you use this record, be aware, as much as you can, of the present-moment-focused "bare attention" that you have been developing through training in mindful awareness. If any questions or observations arise as you practice, write them down so that you might share them with your therapist during your next meeting.

1. **Situation**
   What is going on around you, in your environment, right now? Where are you? Who is with you? What are you doing? What are you noticing in the environment that is affecting you?

2. **Physical Sensations**
   Sometimes our response to something in our environment can be felt in the body, like "butterflies in the stomach," for example. Bringing our attention, as best as we can, to these sensations, can be helpful. Developing awareness and sensitivity to these experiences can take practice, so if you don't notice anything in particular, just allow yourself that experience, while maybe taking a moment or two to give your attention some time to observe whatever may be present. In this situation, what physical sensations do you notice yourself experiencing in your body? Where in your body do you feel such sensations? What are the qualities of such sensations?

3. **Emotions**
   Labeling our emotions using "feeling words" can be helpful. Taking a moment to truly make space for and allow this emotional experience, what "feeling word" would best describe and "label" this emotion that you are feeling in this moment? How intensely would you say you are feeling this emotion? If you

were to rate this emotion on a scale of 0 to 100, with 100 being the most intense feeling you could have, and 0 being no presence of this feeling at all, what would that rating be?

4. Thoughts

What thoughts are going through your mind in this situation? Ask yourself, "What is going through my mind right now? What is my mind telling me?" What is "popping into your head" in this situation? What does this situation say about you? What does this situation suggest about your future? As best as you can, notice the flow of thoughts that unfold in your mind in this situation. What are some of the thoughts that are arriving?

5. "Learning to Stay"

We human beings have learned to try to get rid of, or get away from, things that seem threatening or unpleasant. This makes solid sense when you think about it. As you and your therapist have discussed, attempts to suppress or eliminate distressing thoughts and feeling sometimes makes them much stronger. So, for a moment, take this opportunity to learn to stay with your experience, just as it is. Following the flow of your breath in this moment, as much as you can, make space for whatever unfolds before your mind. In the space below, write down any observations you may make about this simple act of gently making space for your experience, moment by moment.

6. Responding "Inside"

Now that you have noticed, and allowed yourself to more fully experience, the sensations, emotions, and thoughts that have shown up in this situation, how might you best respond in this moment? Adopting a mindful, "emotionally intelligent" attitude, you can recognize that these thoughts and feelings are events in the mind, and not reality itself. Working with your therapist, you can learn many ways to respond to distressing thoughts and feelings. Here are a few questions to ask yourself to practice this week:

"What are the costs and benefits to me of believing these thoughts?"
"How might I act if I really believed this?"
"How might I act if I didn't believe this?"
"What might I say to a friend who was facing this situation?"
"What needs are involved in this event, and how can I best take care of myself now?"
"Can I mindfully observe these events in my mind, choose a course of action, and act in a way that will serve my aims?"
    In the space below, please write your responses and observations.

7. Responding "Outside"

Ask yourself the following questions:

"How can I best pursue my own aims and values in this situation?"
"Is there a problem here that I need to solve in order to live my life in a mean-ingful and valued way?"

"How can I interact with others in this situation in an effective way that suits
  my aims and values?"
"Does this situation call for a behavioral response? Does any action need to
  be taken?
"Is doing nothing an option?"
"How can I take care of myself best in this situation?"

In the space below, please record any responses or observations that involve
ways in which you can use this situation as a step in a life that feels rewarding,
and in tune with your personal values.

Factor 3: Persistence in Awakening (*Viriya-sambojjhaṅga*)

Sometimes translated as "energy," the factor persistence (*viriya*) reflects
the degree to which we can remain committed to the process of awakening to reality and liberation from suffering. This factor involves an
increased engagement with practice, particularly when addressing
unskillful behaviors and experiences of suffering. All behavior change
involves some course correction, mistakes, faltering efforts, and a process of renewal and beginning again. The range of commitment and
behavior change techniques that we find in ACT, DBT, and CBT are
reflections of the factor of persistence. With mindfulness and investigation, we may access perspective and innate wisdom that allow us to
choose how to be in the world. If we are to realize and actualize this
"ability-to-be," then we call upon our persistence of effort, and the
focusing of our will, to follow a disciplined path to our goal. We begin
again as often as the situation requires, persisting or letting go of our
particular behaviors and strategies through the arising factor of persistence of effort and energy. It is telling that this factor can stand for both
persistence and energy. As we practice behavioral activation (Dimidjian
et al., 2006) or the accomplishing of valued aims, the more deeply we
engage in meaningful and rewarding activities, and the more we may
find ourselves experiencing newfound energy and alertness. Commitment and engagement can reverse the constriction and hopelessness of
depression and inactivity. This deeper engagement with living, and the
experience of greater energy, can be like arising from a sleep of rumination, vegetative symptoms, and despondency. As such, we awaken to and
with persistence, and our energy feels restored as we grow more wakeful.

As Thich Nhat Hanh has described, "Even if we are in pain, if we can see meaning in life, we will have energy and joy" (Hanh, 1973, p. 216).

Factor 4: Happiness in Awakening (Pīti-sambojjhaṅga)

Happiness or joyfulness (piti) is the experience of delight. This form of bliss arises when attention is absorbed in a way that is conducive to further movement toward waking up. We are aware that when we are under the aversive control of threat-based emotions, such as anxiety, shame, and anger, our behavioral repertoires become narrower, our attention less flexible, and our choices seem constricted. Perhaps nothing fuels our struggle with avoidance and attachment as much as facing a threatening reality. But we are also hardwired to experience soothing, contentment, perceptual flexibility, and empathy in the presence of positive social emotions and contexts.

According to Barbara Fredrickson's broaden-and-build theory (Frederickson & Branigan, 2005), individuals who experience a higher frequency of positive emotions and positive thinking will be capable of a broader range of responses across the field of functioning. Dimensions of behavior ranging from reaction time to life satisfaction appear to be related to the experience of positive affect (Frederickson & Cohn, 2008). Accordingly, our experience of awakening wisdom and our ensuing capacity to live well involves more than the dominance of cognitive or verbal mediation of behavior, and is situated in our experience of happiness and compassion. It isn't surprising that an intellectual appreciation of the deep interconnectedness of all things would have an emotional dimension. Similarly, when we inhabit the space of feeling soothed, interpersonally connected, and contented, this organizes our minds in such a way that we are much more likely to logically and intellectually apprehend the illusion of separateness. Perhaps happiness is involved in awakening because the natural selection of genetic variations has led to the enlightenment experience feeling reinforcing. Then again, perhaps this is simply the happiness of our truly and finally coming home again.

Factor 5: Serenity in Awakening (Passaddhi-sambojjhaṅga)

Freedom of action in our thoughts, feelings, and behaviors is often accompanied by an experience of calm and centeredness that may be described as serenity. The fifth factor, serenity (*passaddhi*), involves the calming, focusing, and stilling of body and mind.

As we have noted, our experience in social emotions and the activation of our contentment system involves a blend of physical relaxation, connectedness, a sense of social safeness, and contentment (Gilbert, 2009a). According to the teachings of the seven factors of awakening, consistent practice of deep meditation and the Eightfold Path will help us to activate an experience of tranquility and ease. This experience of serenity can create the proper context for our subsequent deeper engagement in the process of awakening and personal evolution. An obvious connection between this fifth factor and the current aims of the cognitive and behavioral therapies is cultivating an ability to meet our experiences of stress, anxiety, and strain with greater mindfulness, willingness, and compassion for self and others. Much of the stress in our lives stems from an experience of social isolation, worries that we won't be able to meet the demands of our lives, and a general overabundance of distractions and pressures. As tragic as the experience of life on earth may be, most of our day-to-day stressors are not actually matters of life or death. Nevertheless, our evolved threat detection system and our inborn and ingrained tendencies toward avoidance and overcompensation can provoke internal and external responses that are essentially based in our survival mechanisms rather than actual, present life-or-death contingencies. The factors of the awakened mind allow us to mindfully make contact with the present moment, investigate the nature and function of our mental events, commit to persistent engagement with meaningful and life-sustaining behaviors, and open ourselves to the joy that may arise in the present moment through our gradual awakening. The next step in this logical sequence is an experience of serenity and calm that proceeds from our happiness and joyfulness. Just as our experience of social contentment biologically evokes a sense of safeness, the fourth factor of awakening, happiness, proceeds to a place of serenity that cultivates a transcendent wisdom and a deep and abiding experience of compassion for all sentient beings.

Concentration in Awakening (*Samādhi-sambojjhaṅga*)

Concentration (*samadhi*) involves settling and composing the mind and focusing it with pointed attention to the present moment. The focus in the experience of *samadhi* (sometimes translated as meditative suspension) is on the unification of those processes involved in awareness and attention, as described in the sections on healthy concentration on the Eightfold Path in Chapter 4. Conventional Western understanding of concentration involves fine-tuning our awareness on some object, which is usually outside of ourselves. The two linguistic components of the Sanskrit word for concentration represent a bringing-together of the energy of the mind, rather than an external focus. In concentration meditation practice, such as Zen meditation, the practitioner collects the attention and resources of the mind consciously and aims it toward an object of focus. Quite often this point of focus is on the breath. In time, the practice of bringing one's pointed concentration to our various mental experiences can help to cultivate our ability to sustain present-centered awareness, and a calming of the discursiveness of our minds. Importantly, this quieting of the mind does not occur through suppression of experience, but through many iterations of practice in gently and compassionately redirecting potential resources and holding such resources in a disciplined, relaxed focus.

Importantly, Buddhist scholars such as Thich Nhat Hanh (1973) point out that cultivating concentration is not an end in itself. In the early 2000s one of us [D. T.] conducted a form of group therapy for PTSD that involved teaching heavy combat veterans both mindfulness and concentration meditation (Tirch & Amodio, 2006). A number of the veterans reported that the experience of concentration meditation reminded them of the sustained focus that they had learned to deploy when they were involved in sniper missions. So, we can see that concentration, like many of the factors of enlightenment and aspects of Buddhist psychology, does not have an inherent ethical or psychological value divorced from its application. It is when concentration is developed in coordination with the other components of the awakened mind, and the motivation to alleviate the suffering that we encounter in the world and ourselves, that this factor of awakening contributes to an enhancement of wisdom, compassion, and overall well-being. At least, this is the position we find in Buddhism. For this to be tested, psychologists will need to frame scientific hypotheses and conduct research. Nevertheless, as we have seen, a substantial body of process research supports such a position, and suggests that the cultivation of what Buddhist psychology would describe as wholesome states can contribute to an ongoing enhancement of our mental and physical health, and perhaps some experience akin to what the *dharma* describes as awakening.

Factor 7: Equanimity in Awakening (*Upekkhā-sambojjhaṅga*)

Equanimity (*upekkha*) or the balance and nonreactivity of mind is the seventh factor of awakening. This feeling state is described as sublime, satisfying, and fulfilling. Again, elements of this state are similar to the feeling state of contentment that is associated with secure attachment and the safeness-based emotion regulation system, (Gilbert, 2009a) known as the affliliatve system. Equanimity reflects the awakening wisdom of our knowledge that everything remains intimately connected, equal, and impermanent. Equanimity reflects an acceptance that this is how things are, and by extension, everything is as it should be. Accordingly, equanimity involves openness to experience in a nonclinging, nondefensive manner. *Upekkha* is also sometimes translated as involving an act of letting go. Seeing all things as equal and interconnected, we may seem to be neutral or indifferent to life. However, this is not the aim or the outcome of the process of developing equanimity. Far from such abandonment of care and connection, *upekkha* involves the wisdom and compassion that comes from viewing all beings, and in fact all phenomena, as a part of ourselves. When we see ourselves in all things, and we are moved by the suffering and joy of living experience itself, our emotions extend into a place of loving-kindness, sympathetic joy, and warm regard for the act of being in a nonpersonal and truly transcendent way. In this way, the seventh factor of awakening opens the door for a much broader experience of being alive.

CASE FORMULATION, THE EIGHTFOLD PATH, AND WAKING UP

The material we have presented on the factors of awakening is drawn from a tradition that holds a particular point of view on what we human beings have the potential to accomplish through mental training. This chapter provides perspectives upon the concept of enlightenment that correlate in cognitive and behavioral psychologies, and that relate to workable aspects of CBT. Of course, many of the philosophical assertions and positions that are outlined here may seem strange to many CBT practitioners. Then again, given how popular acceptance- and compassion-based therapies have become, perhaps this is familiar territory for many of our readers.

Regardless of the potential newness of the concepts, or the expansive nature of some of the aims of Buddhist psychology, when we look closely at the assumptions underlying them, we find that little is being taken for granted. As the Dalai Lama has repeatedly said, if science should disprove any part of Buddhism, then Buddhism should be changed. Much like a traditional Buddhist practitioner, cognitive-behavioral therapists would be well advised to take none of the above on faith. Rather, any person seeking to apply the Middle Path intervention, or indeed any of the range of Buddhist practices, to their psychotherapy or personal growth, is better off treating all of the teachings he or she encounters as hypotheses to be tested.

In terms of case formulation, these ideas from Buddhist psychology provide us with a number of new variables that can be dealt with in CBT. When we conduct workshops, participants often ask us how we might best know which diagnosis or cluster of symptoms is the best match for a particular form of meditation, imagery, or other Buddhist psychology-based practice. Rather than leaping to equating particular diagnostic classifications with specific aspects of Buddhist mental training, we suggest taking a *dharma*-informed functional and dimensional approach to adding Buddhist psychology to your CBT case formulation and treatment development.

Throughout the text, several techniques and concepts have been linked, and are related to certain areas of human functioning. In order to apply this material to your current case conceptualization, you might ask yourself a series of questions about your client, and aim to answer them from a place of mindfulness, willingness, and compassion. We hope that, having developed your own personal practice, and also having formulated a CBT case conceptualization consistent with whatever form of therapy with which you are working (ACT, DBT, CT, etc.), you might choose to deploy some mindfulness, slowing down and asking yourself a series of questions as we did at the beginning of this book.

The Middle Path Formulation

To begin, gather your attention as you have been practicing through training in mindfulness, concentration, compassion, or any of the range of contemplative practices available to you. Bring yourself into the present moment and rest in the breath. When the mind moves into distraction and inevitable wandering, gently and persistently bring yourself back to this moment, as you have learned to do through practice. When you find this attention collected, bring your client to mind. Recall your emotional experiences and observations when working with this client, and allow yourself to empathically bridge into his or her experience.

From this place of mindful awareness and access to your own compassionate wisdom, ask yourself the following questions, and record your observations, either by writing down your responses or by recording them with an audio application. This is a practice of mindful and intentional case formulation, not an eyes-closed exercise. As much as the practice is for your client, and aimed at targeting areas to develop strength, your engagement in the practice is for you, and for the furtherance of our shared aim: the alleviation of the suffering we experience in others and ourselves, and perhaps even to wake up to the wisdom and compassion of our awakened minds.

The questions follow:

• **First Noble Truth:** When remembering the Four Noble Truths, how much do you think this client has realized and begun to accept that suffering is a part of life for us all? How much does this sense of common humanity and the shared struggle of life reach the client? How does the client relate to suffering?

• **Second Noble Truth:** To what degree does this person realize that patterns of avoidance and obsessive craving are driving much of his or her suffering? How much does he or she recognize that his or her efforts to excessively avoid or control suffering are harmful—that the solution is the problem? What are the person's patterns of nonacceptance and excessive attachment to imaginary outcomes?

• **Third Noble Truth:** To what extent does this person recognize that while pain is inevitable, to some degree suffering is optional? How much is this client willing to entertain the idea that if we let go of our patterns of avoidance and excessive craving, we can move in meaningful directions in our lives that can lead to the cessation of suffering? How willing is the client to let go of the struggle and try something new? What might this look like for him or her?

• **Fourth Noble Truth—The Middle Path:** In the service of living a life that moves toward greater realization and meaning and away from a cycle of suffering and struggle, how willing and capable is this person to engage in new patterns of action? What might these patterns look like? What strengths does this person possess that will help him or her in this process? What obstacles might he or she find in moving toward

  ▪ **Healthy Speech:** Speaking their truth and communicating healthily, with others and with themselves, from a place of clarity, purpose, and honesty?

  ▪ **Healthy Action:** Engaging in healthy actions that serve to promote the well-being of themselves and others, without creating needless suffering?

  ▪ **Healthy Livelihood:** Supporting themselves and earning their livelihood in ways that contribute to a healthy state of mind and body, promoting life-sustaining, wise, and compassionate aims for self and others?

  ▪ **Healthy Effort:** Maintaining a healthy and sustained effort to live life in a balanced and self-nurturing way that returns in kindness to the pursuit of the cessation of suffering and promotion of wellness for self and others?

- **Healthy Mindfulness:** Cultivating and maintaining flexible and focused attention to the present moment with acceptance, curiosity, and kindness?

- **Healthy Concentration:** Gathering and concentrating their attention and guided awareness to maintain sustained focus in a one-pointed way?

- **Healthy Intention:** Choosing to maintain an adaptive relationship to thoughts, emotions, and actions that focuses on the alleviation of suffering and the promotion of well-being and awakening to the nature of things?

- **Healthy Understanding:** Developing a deeper understanding of the nature of the mind, the self, and our relationship to the world around us, in the service of cultivating wisdom, compassion and living a meaningful and purposeful life?

To what extent might this person be able to consciously develop the following qualities in the service of a deliberate development of wisdom, compassion, skillful means, and an expanding realization of what it means to be a living being, for the person's own good and the good of those around him or her? What are his or her strengths and areas for growth in terms of the **Seven Factors of Awakening**?

• **Awakening Mindfulness:** Paying attention in the present moment with acceptance, purpose, and nonjudgment of his or her experience.

• **Awakening Analysis:** Bringing a wise and rational perspective to his or her moment-by-moment experience, and balancing his or her emotional responses, valued aims, logical thinking, and innate sense of knowing what is true and right to form new perspectives.

• **Awakening Persistence:** Maintaining committed and persistent effort and healthily tending to his or her emotional and physical resources, in pursuit of alleviation of suffering.

• **Awakening Happiness:** Being open to positive emotional experiences and allowing a sense of joyfulness and healthy positive emotions to serve as a compass in moving toward greater wisdom and wellness for self and others.

• **Awakening Serenity:** Accessing and realizing an experience of calmness, tranquility, and relaxation in the course of life; bringing an experience of release, softening, and gentleness into contact with unnecessary tensions.

• **Awakening Concentration:** Intentionally developing his or her ability for sustained attention and dis-identification with the flow of his or her thinking, in the service of realizing a deeper knowledge and experience of what it means to be human.

• **Awakening Equanimity:** Cultivating a balanced and open view of all living things as elements of a broader, universal context of interconnectedness, impermanence, and countless cause-and-effect connections across reality—and gently accepting the nature of living as it presents itself with self-compassion and a balanced mind.

Elements of the two psychologies of compassion are:

• **Compassionate Engagement and Awareness:** To what degree does this client feel sensitive to the suffering he or she experience in self and others, and to what degree is he or she able to turn toward the suffering they encounter in the world?

• **Compassionate Alleviation and Prevention:** To what degree does this client experience a motivation to do something to alleviate and prevent the suffering he or she encounters in him- or herself and others?

We have included a case formulation that one of us completed in working with Rita, whom we met early in this book, as an example of the kind of information and treatment directions that might be generated through a Buddhist-informed CBT understanding of our clients. Importantly, the case conceptualization was completed from a deliberate place of mindful compassion, and represents a coming together of our analytic capacity with our deliberate focus on mindfulness, acceptance, compassion, and inner wisdom.

The Middle Path Case Formulation for Rita

First Noble Truth: When remembering the Four Noble Truths, how much do you think this client has realized and begun to accept that suffering is a part of life for us all? How much does this sense of common humanity and the shared struggle of life reach him or her? How does the client relate to suffering?

Initially Rita felt she was the only one who suffered like she did and that she deserved her pain and suffering. She would make comments like "evidence-based therapies won't work for someone like me." In addition to initially blaming herself for her suffering and expressing a sense that she deserved it, Rita would also shame and harshly criticize herself for her pain and suffering.

Second Noble Truth: To what degree does this person realize that patterns of avoidance and obsessive craving are driving much of his or her suffering? What are his or her patterns of nonacceptance and excessive attachment to imaginary outcomes? What are his or her go-to avoidance, control, or safety behaviors? How much does he or she recognize that his or her efforts to excessively avoid or control suffering are harmful—that the solution is the problem?

Rita tried to avoid her experiences of PTSD and panic attacks through many different methods, such as drinking, compulsive exercising, antidepressants, isolation, checking behaviors, and not leaving her apartment. She came to therapy with a sense of unworkability in her prior attempts to "get rid of" her PTSD. She spoke of how not leaving her apartment and ignoring relationships have made her "pathetic" and that she couldn't be "normal." Early on in treatment Rita had a mixed set of beliefs around her efforts for control and avoidance as problematic and, at the same time, beneficial and necessary. However, she found a sense of relief or validation in the idea that perhaps she couldn't avoid or get rid of her suffering, and that her prior attempts at control may not have been much benefit at all and only made her life feel even smaller and her options more limited.

Third Noble Truth: To what extent does this person recognize that while pain is inevitable, to some degree suffering is optional? How much is this client willing to entertain the idea that if we let go of our patterns of avoidance and excessive craving, we can move in meaningful directions in our lives that can lead to the cessation of suffering? How willing is the client to let go of the struggle and try something new? What might this look like for him or her?

While Rita came to view her attempts to avoid and get rid of pain and suffering as futile in a relatively short time in therapy, she struggled with an initial willingness to let these go and try something new. She had been so disappointed in treatment and other attempts to change in the past that she was skeptical of therapy being able to help her. She also reported frustration with feeling stuck in the belief that "nothing works for me" and at the same time scared that this belief would always be true. By accessing some of her values and clarifying her desired outcomes, Rita was able to see that new behaviors might keep her struggle and suffering from immobilizing her, and making her feel stuck. She began to see her process of letting go of the struggle as "relearning to live my life." This process of Rita "taking my life back" included values and goals clarification, compassionate exposure, and mindfulness of thoughts and emotions, and was aided by the development of an ideal compassionate image to help or coach her through the process of changing avoidance and control patterns

Fourth Noble Truth—The Middle Path: In the service of living a life that moves toward greater realization and meaning and away from a cycle of suffering and struggle, how willing and capable is this person to engage in new patterns of action? What might these patterns look like? What strengths do they possess that will help him or her in this process? What obstacles might he or she find in moving toward:

Healthy Speech: Speaking their truth and communicating healthily, with others and with themselves, from a place of clarity, purpose and honesty?

OBSTACLES: *Initially, Rita was not very willing to speak to many people; she was isolating and avoiding conversations with strangers, acquaintances, friends, and family. When she did speak with someone she would often speak from a place of anger and frustration or self-deprecation. When it came to speaking to herself, Rita was quite harsh and critical, calling herself "stupid," "pathetic," or a "loser." The tone of this self-talk was one of anger, frustration, contempt, and disappointment. She blamed and condemned herself and often reminded herself that she deserved her suffering.*

STRENGTHS: *When it came to healthy speech Rita was able to access an ability to communicate effectively with the therapist and often spoke from a place of authenticity with an aim of honesty.*

Healthy Action: Engaging in healthy actions that serve to promote the well-being of him- or herself and others, without creating needless suffering?

OBSTACLES: *Rita had a long history and patterns of avoidance. She had many years of drinking and was regularly smoking cigarettes when she entered therapy. She had been an avid exercise enthusiast in the past and reported "like many things I do, I took it to the extreme, and injured my knee, ankle, and shoulder."*

STRENGTHS: *Rita valued healthy eating and nutrition, she loved to garden and grow her own vegetables, and she prepared healthy meals for herself (and in the past for others).*

Healthy Livelihood: Supporting themselves and earning their livelihood in ways that contribute to a healthy state of mind and body, promoting life-sustaining, wise, and compassionate aims for self and others?

OBSTACLES: *Rita was unemployed when she entered treatment. She had left her job due to overwhelming experiences of anxiety and panic at work. She was currently living off of support from her family. She describes herself as a perfectionist and workaholic who "never got close to perfect." When she was working or in graduate school, she prioritized work above all else, at the sacrifice of friendships, sleep, or hobbies/recreation.*

STRENGTHS: *Prior to leaving work, Rita was employed as an adjunct biology professor. She had received her PhD and considered herself to be an excellent student and she loves to learn new things and to teach others.*

Healthy Effort: Maintaining a healthy and sustained effort to live life in a balanced and self-nurturing way, that returns in kindness to the pursuit of the cessation of suffering and promotion of wellness for self and others?

OBSTACLES: *Rita is a self-described perfectionist and workaholic. She says she will do whatever she can to avoid failure and often takes any project, interest, or responsibility to the "extreme." She denies herself "pleasure or reward" if she feels she has failed or come close to failing and often is harsh, critical, and punishing of any "laziness."*

STRENGTHS: *Rita reported that she always felt a deep desire to let herself have a "well-balanced life" and that she has always encouraged others to work as hard and play as hard as they feel is good for them. However, she says she has historically found it impossible to give herself permission to do the same.*

Healthy Mindfulness: Cultivating and maintaining flexible and focused attention to the present moment with acceptance, curiosity, and kindness?

OBSTACLES: *Rita was very skeptical and wary of mindfulness, particularly given her experiences of flashbacks and intrusive health anxiety and panic. She was reportedly very good at multitasking, autopilot, and getting through certain tasks or experiences as quickly as possible. She viewed herself as a taskmaster constantly pushing herself to hurry up and also as her personal judge and jury relentlessly evaluating and scrutinizing her performance or her current state of safety or health and well-being.*

STRENGTHS: *Rita had some understanding of the principles of mindfulness and found that she did have some mindfulness experiences in gardening and prior mediation training.*

Healthy Concentration: Gathering and concentrating their attention and guided awareness to maintain sustained focus in a one-pointed way?

OBSTACLES: *Given her tendency toward multitasking and avoidance of intrusive or painful experiences or memories, healthy concentration was a reported challenge for Rita. She would often avoid any task that required sustained attention for fear of unwanted experiences. She also avoided one-pointed concentration as she just "knows I am going to suck at it and fail, again."*

STRENGTHS: *Rita could appreciate the value in healthy concentration and had this ability in the past. She reportedly longed for the days back in grad school when she was able to sit in the library and read and attend to a single book or journal article.*

Healthy Intention: Choosing to maintain an adaptive relationship to thoughts, emotions, and actions that focuses on the alleviation of suffering and the promotion of well-being and awakening to the nature of things?

OBSTACLES: When Rita entered therapy she often responded to herself with contempt and used punishment rather than reinforcement. She would hold herself accountable for all failings or mistakes and use harsh responses to her private and public events and experiences. In particular, she would criticize and blame herself for perceived mistakes and an inability to escape her PTSD and anxiety experiences.

STRENGTHS: When it came to healthy intentions for others, Rita revealed a strong capacity for encouragement, support, and kindness. She displayed perspective-taking abilities and appeared to be able to see what others did well and then consider constructive, helpful learning points, particularly in her graduate school peers and student with whom she had worked for as a professor.

Healthy Understanding: Developing a deeper understanding of the nature of the mind, the self, and our relationship to the world around us, in the service of cultivating wisdom, compassion, and living a meaningful and purposeful life?

OBSTACLES: Rita entered therapy with a strong and well-rehearsed negative bias toward herself and her future. She reported that she was hopeless and fully to blame.

STRENGTHS: Rita expressed a strong desire to be more aware and effective in her understanding of herself, her world, and her life. She was willing to entertain new and different worldviews and was constantly seeking out new, effective points for understanding herself and others.

The Seven Factors of Awakening: To what extent might this person be able to consciously develop the following qualities in the service of a deliberate development of wisdom, compassion, skillful means, and an expanding realization of what it means to be a living being, for his or her own good and the good of those around him or her? What are his or her strengths and areas for growth in terms of—(Awakening Mindfulness) Paying attention in the present moment with acceptance, purpose, and nonjudgment of their experience?

Rita has demonstrated a growing capacity to contact the present moment in her initial mindfulness practice and in her gentle yoga practice.

(Awakening Analysis) Bringing a wise and rational perspective to his or her moment-by-moment experience, and balancing his or her emotional responses, valued aims, logical thinking, and innate sense of knowing what is true and right to form new perspectives?

Rita has a keen intelligence and a capacity to be rational. She can, however, become entangled in rumination and worry when she avoids feeling states and direct contingencies to focus on logic and rationality alone.

(Awakening Persistence) Maintaining committed and persistent effort and healthily tending to his or her emotional and physical resources, in pursuit of alleviation of suffering?

Despite her ability to remain persistent in her academic pursuits, Rita has had a historic difficulty in maintaining persistence and committed action when she is motivated to alleviate and prevent her own suffering, or to face challenging emotional states in the service of personal growth.

(Awakening Happiness) Being open to positive emotional experiences and allowing a sense of joyfulness and healthy positive emotions to serve as a compass in moving toward greater wisdom and wellness for self and others

This client's emotional avoidance has not only been limited to negative emotions. Her painful attachment history and social learning has led her to sometimes experience threat emotions that are triggered by the presence of positive emotions. As such, gradual exposure to allowing herself to experience positive affect is indicated.

(Awakening Concentration) Intentionally developing his or her ability for sustained attention and dis-identification with the flow of his or her thinking, in the service of realizing a deeper knowledge and experience of what it means to be human?

The client has a capacity for sustained attention when engaged with stimulating material, and when involved in emotional avoidance. However, ongoing training in developing flexible, focused attention that can serve to cultivate a capacity for concentration and equanimity would be useful.

(Awakening Equanimity) Cultivating a balanced and open view of all living things as elements of a broader, universal context of interconnectedness, impermanence, and countless cause-and-effect connections across reality—and—gently accepting the nature of living as it presents itself with self-compassion and a balanced mind?

Rita has a great capacity to be nonjudgmental and compassionately noncondemning with others and with animals. However, her self-judgmental thoughts and chronic experience of shame makes it difficult for her to maintain a noncondemning perspective on her own experiences or on herself.

To what degree does this client feel sensitive to the suffering he or she experiences in self and others, and to what degree is he or she able to turn toward the suffering he or she encounters in the world? (Compassionate Engagement and Awareness)

Rita's capacity for present-moment-focused sensitivity is a potential strength, and her sympathetic reaction to notice and be moved by suffering is high. However, the client struggles to find the willingness needed to turn toward her fear and her pain and engage with this material.

To what degree does this client experience a motivation to do something to alleviate and prevent the suffering he or she encounters in him- or herself and others? (Compassionate Alleviation and Prevention)

Rita is highly motivated to alleviate and prevent her suffering. However, her persistent patterns of avoidance and struggling to change chronically occurring inner experiences has made it difficult for her to translate this motivation into action.

Based on how you respond to the questions on pages 217–219, you might wish to reflect on what dimensions of a Buddhist psychology-informed treatment might benefit from greater attention over the course of the therapy. For example, a patient who has great difficulty maintaining a mindful perspective might benefit from more training in this area in order to facilitate his or her openness to difficult emotions during exposure and response prevention. Conversely, an individual with stubborn patterns of behavioral avoidance and procrastination might benefit from cultivating concentration and self-compassion, as well as building his or her capacity for healthy effort and awakening persistence. You might wish to share some of these observations with your client in the course of collaborative case formulation and treatment planning. Importantly, this case formulation is meant to augment and supplement the evidence-based intervention that forms the center of your work with the client. No outcome research of therapy specifically designed through such a formulation exists. However, we have been careful to outline the supporting process research and provide techniques to support a Buddhist psychology-informed CBT throughout the text, with each intervention linked to potentially meaningful and effective processes. For some clients, symptom remission, and perhaps even living more values-driven lives may not be enough. Some may benefit from connecting their lives to a motivation to alleviate the suffering they encounter and develop a gradual awakening to a wisdom of how things are, and who they are. This may not be every client, and yet many may relate to this deeper motivation. Additionally, processes such as compassion, acceptance, mindfulness, and the elements of the Eightfold Path are useful in the alleviation of suffering even for those who don't know precisely what they are seeking. Like the original meaning of *Dukkha*, the feeling of a wheel out of balance, the only requirement to begin a path toward freedom from suffering and waking up to reality is a knowledge that something is wrong—and a motivation to do something about it.

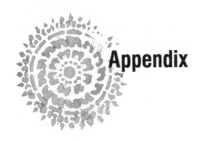 **Appendix**

Foundational Elements
of Buddhist Psychology

Below we have provided a brief list of the foundational elements of Buddhist psychology. With so many of the central ideas in Buddhist psychology having been described in the form of enumerated lists, keeping all of these components in order can be a bit challenging. Conversely, when one can easily call to mind the various units of the system, such as "the seven factors of awakening," the range of different phenomena and concepts can be more readily brought to mind, and used in case conceptualization and interventions. The glossary below is meant to serve as a reference as you integrate an understanding of Buddhist psychology into your knowledge and practice of CBT.

Bodhi: enlightenment, awakening.

Bodhicitta: a spontaneously arising aspiration for awakening, and for the cessation of suffering of all sentient beings.

Bodhisattva: a person who is on the path toward enlightenment, and who commits all of their lives to the cessation of suffering and enlightenment of all sentient beings, even at the cost of delaying their own enlightenment and liberation from suffering.

Brahmaviharas: four "immeasurable qualities"—(1) *karuna* (compassion); (2) *metta* (loving-kindness); (3) *mudita* (sympathetic joy); and (4) *upeekha* (equanimity).

Dharma: Universal laws and cosmic order. Also used to describe the teachings of Buddhism.

First Noble Truth: *dukkha*; CBT practice: conditioned reality, self, and suffering.

Four foundations of mindfulness: (1) *kaya-sati*: mindfulness of the body; (2) *vedana-sati*: mindfulness of feelings; (3) *citta-sati*: mindfulness of the mind or consciousness; and (4) *dhamma-sati*: mindfulness of mental phenomena.

Fourth Noble Truth: the Middle Path—the eightfold process to liberation: adaptive conduct (healthy speech, healthy action, healthy livelihood); mental discipline (healthy effort, healthy mindfulness, healthy concentration); and wisdom (healthy intention, healthy understanding).

Karma: "cause and effect"; action and consequence particularly as refers to how an individual's actions and intentions will influence their future experience.

Prajna paramita: perfection of transcendent wisdom.

Second Noble Truth: the origin of suffering; CBT practice: learning theory, experiential avoidance.

Seven factors for awakening (*bojjhaṅga*): (1) mindfulness in awakening (*sati-sambojjhaṅga*); (2) investigation in awakening (*dhamma-vicaya-sambojjhaṅga*); (3) persistence in awakening (*viriya-sambojjhaṅga*); (4) happiness in awakening (*pīti-sambojjhaṅga*); (5) serenity in awakening (*passaddhi-sambojjhaṅga*); (6) concentration in awakening (*samādhi-sambojjhaṅga*); and (7) equanimity in awakening (*upekkhā-sambojjhaṅga*).

Shunyata: emptiness.

Third Noble Truth: liberation from suffering; CBT practice: creative hopelessness, motivational interviewing.

Three marks of existence: (1) impermanence; (2) no-self; (3) suffering.

Two Truths: a philosophy or doctrine in Buddhism that describes two levels of truth being experienced by humans. The first, relative truth, describes our experience of a concrete and predictable world and of the separateness of individual and environment. The second, absolute truth, describes a state of limitless potentiality for all things, devoid of separateness or inherent existence.

References

Abramowitz, J. S., Tolin, D. F., & Street, G. P. (2001). Paradoxical effects of thought suppression: A meta-analysis of controlled studies. *Clinical Psychology Review, 21*, 683–703.

Adele, M. H., & Feldman, G. (2004). Clarifying the construct of mindfulness in the context of emotion regulation and the process of change in therapy. *Clinical Psychology, 11*, 255–262.

Alexander, C. N., Robinson, P., Orme-Johnson, D. W., Schneider, R. H., & Walton, K. G. (1994). The effects of transcendental meditation compared to other methods of relaxation and meditation in reducing risk factors, morbidity, and mortality. *Homeostasis, 35*, 243–263.

Alford, B. A., & Beck, A. T. (1998). *The integrative power of cognitive therapy.* New York: Guilford Press.

Allen, N. B., & Knight, W. E. J. (2005). Mindfulness, compassion for self, and compassion for others: Implications for understanding the psychopathology and treatment of depression. In P. Gilbert (Ed.), *Compassion: Conceptualisations, research and use in psychotherapy* (pp. 239–262). London: Routledge.

Allen, R. E. (1959). Anamnesis in Plato's "Meno and Phaedo." *Review of Metaphysics, 13*, 165–174.

Allman, J. M., Hakeem, A., Erwin, J. M., Nimchinsky, E., & Hof, P. (2001). The anterior cingulate cortex: The evolution of an interface between emotion and cognition. *Annals of the New York Academy of Science, 935*(1), 107–117.

Anderson, N. D., Lau, M. A., Segal, Z. V., & Bishop, S. R. (2007). Mindfulness-based stress reduction and attentional control. *Clinical Psychology and Psychotherapy, 14*(6), 449–463.

Arch, J. J., & Craske, M. G. (2006). Mechanisms of mindfulness: Emotion regulation following a focused breathing instruction. *Behavior Research and Therapy, 44*, 1849–1858.

Astin, J. (1997). Stress reduction through mindfulness meditation: Effects in psychological symptomatology, sense of control and spiritual experiences. *Psychotherapy and Psychosomatics, 66*(2), 97–106.

Atkins, P., & Parker, S. (2011). Understanding individual compassion in organizations: The role of appraisals and psychological flexibility. *Academy of Management Review, 37*(4), 524–546.

Atkinson, A. P., & Wheeler, M. (2003). Evolutionary psychology's brain problem and the cognitive neuroscience of reasoning. In D. Over (Ed.), *Evolution and the psychology of thinking: The debate* (pp. 61–99). Hove, UK: Psychology Press.

Austin, J. H. (1999). *Zen and the brain: Toward an understanding of meditation and consciousness.* Cambridge, MA: MIT Press.

Baer, R. A. (2003). Mindfulness training as a clinical intervention: A conceptual and empirical review. *Clinical Psychology: Science and Practice, 10,* 125–143.

Baer, R. A. (2009). Self-focused attention and mechanisms of change in mindfulness-based treatment. *Cognitive Behaviour Therapy, 38,* 15–20.

Baker, L. R., & McNulty, J. K. (2011). Self-compassion and relationship maintenance: The moderating roles of conscientiousness and gender. *Journal of Personality and Social Psychology, 100*(5), 853–873.

Baker, T. B., McFall, R. M., & Shoham, V. (2009). Current status and future prospects of clinical psychology: Toward a scientifically principled approach to mental and behavioral health care. *Association for Psychological Science: Journal of the Association of Psychological Science, 9,* 67–103.

Barley, W. D., Buie, S. E., Peterson, E. W., Hollingsworth, A. S., Griva, M., Hickerson, S. C., et al. (1993). Development of an inpatient cognitive-behavioral treatment program for borderline personality disorder. *Journal of Personality Disorders, 7*(3), 232–240.

Barlow, D. H. (2004). *Anxiety and its disorders: The nature and treatment of anxiety and panic* (2nd ed.). New York: Guilford Press.

Barnard, L. K., & Curry, J. F. (2011). Self-compassion: Conceptualizations, correlates, and interventions. *Review of General Psychology, 15,* 289–303.

Barnes, S., Brown, K. W., Krusemark, E., Campbell, W. K., & Rogge, R. D. (2007). The role of mindfulness in romantic relationship satisfaction and responses to relationship stress. *Journal of Marital and Family Therapy, 33*(4), 482–500.

Barnes-Holmes, Y., Hayes, S.C., Barnes-Holmes, D., & Roche, B. (2002). Relational frame theory: A post-Skinnerian account of human language and cognition. *Advances in Childhood Development and Behavior, 28,* 101–138.

Bartels, A., & Zeki, S. (2004). The neural correlates of maternal and romantic love. *NeuroImage, 21,* 1155–1166.

Beck, A. T. (1970). *Depression: Causes and treatment.* New York: Harper & Row.

Beck, A. T. (1976). *Cognitive therapy and the emotional disorders.* New York: Meridian.

Beck, A. T. (2008). The evolution of the cognitive model of depression and its neurobiological correlates. *American Journal of Psychiatry, 165*(8), 969–977.

Beck, A. T., & Clark, D. A. (1988). Anxiety and depression: An information processing perspective. *Anxiety Research, 1*(1), 23–36.

Beck, A. T., Rush, A. J., Shaw, B. F., & Emery, G. (1979). *Cognitive therapy of depression.* New York: Guilford Press.

Becker, D. E., & Shapiro, D. (1981). Physiological responses to clicks during Zen, yoga, and TM. *Psychophysiology, 18,* 694–699.

Beer, R. (2003). *The handbook of Tibetan Buddhist symbols.* Boston: Shambhala.

Bein, A. (2008). *The Zen of helping: Spiritual principles for mindful and openhearted practice.* Hoboken, NJ: Wiley.

Bein, T. (2010). *The Buddha's way of happiness.* Oakland, CA: New Harbinger.

Beitel, M., Ferrer, E., & Cerero, J. J. (2005). Psychological mindedness and awareness of self and others. *Journal of Clinical Psychology, 61,* 739–750.

Bernstein, S. S. (2003). Positive organizational scholarship: Meet the movement. An interview with Kim Cameron, Jane Dutton, and Robert Quinn. *Journal of Management Inquiry, 12,* 266–271.

Birnie, K., Speca, M., & Carlson, L. E. (2010). Exploring self-compassion and empathy in the context of mindfulness-based stress reduction (MBSR). *Stress and Health, 26*(5), 359–371.

Bishop, S. R. (2002). What do we really know about mindfulness-based stress reduction? *Psychosomatic Medicine, 64,* 71–84.

Bishop, S. R., Lau, M., Shapiro, S., Carlson, L., Anderson, N. D., Carmody, J. C., et al. (2004). Mindfulness: A proposed operational definition. *Clinical Psychology: Science and Practice, 11,* 230–241.

Bodhi, B. (Ed.). (2000a). *Abhidhammatha Sangaha: A comprehensive manual of Abhidhamma.* Onalaska, WA: Buddhist Psychology/S. Pariyatti.

Bodhi, B. (2000b). *A comprehensive manual of Adhidhamma.* Seattle, WA: Buddhist Psychology/S. Pariyatti.

Bodhi, B. (Trans.). (2000c). *The connected discourses of the Buddha: A translation of the* Samyutta Nikaya. Somerville, MA: Wisdom.

Bodhi, B. (2005). *In the Buddha's words: An anthology of discourses from the Pali Canon.* Somerville, MA: Wisdom.

Bodhi, B., & Nanamoli, B. (Eds. & Trans.). (1995). *The middle length discourses of the Buddha: A new translation of the* Majjhima Nikaya. Somerville, MA: Wisdom.

Bonanno, G. A., Papa, A., Lalande, K., Westphal, M., & Coifman, K. (2004). The importance of being flexible: The ability to both enhance and suppress emotional expression predicts long-term adjustment. *Psychological Science, 15,* 482–487.

Borkovec, T. D., & Roemer, L. (1995). Perceived functions of worry among generalized anxiety disorder subjects: Distraction from more emotionally distressing topics? *Journal of Behavior Therapy and Experimental Psychiatry, 26,* 25–30.

Bowen, S., Chawla, N., Collins, S. E., Witkiewitz, K., Hsu, S., Grow, J., et al. (2009). Mindfulness-based relapse prevention for substance use disorders: A pilot efficacy trial. *Substance Abuse, 30*(4), 295–305.

Bowen, S., Chawla, N., & Marlatt, G. A. (2011). *Mindfulness-based relapse prevention for addictive behaviors: A clinician's guide*. New York: Guilford Press.

Brown, K. W., & Cordon, S. (2009). Toward a phenomenology of mindfulness: Subjective experience and emotional correlates. In F. Didonna (Ed.), *The clinical handbook of mindfulness* (pp. 59–81). New York: Springer.

Brown, K. W., & Gerbarg, P. L. (2012). *The healing power of breath*. Boston: Shambhala.

Brown, K. W., & Ryan, R. M. (2003). The benefits of being present: Mindfulness and its role in psychological well-being. *Journal of Personality and Social Psychology, 84*, 822–848.

Brown, K. W., & Ryan, R. M. (2004). Perils and promise in defining and measuring mindfulness: Observations from experience. *Clinical Psychology Science and Practice, 11*, 242–248.

Brown, K. W., Ryan, R. M., & Creswell, C. D. (2007). Mindfulness: Theoretical foundations and evidence for its salutary effects. *Psychological Inquiry, 18*, 211–237.

Buss, D. M. (1995). Evolutionary psychology: A new paradigm for psychological science. *Psychological Inquiry, 6*, 1–49.

Butler, A. C., Chapman, J. E., Forman, E. M., & Beck, A. T. (2006). The empirical status of cognitive-behavioral therapy: A review of meta-analyses. *Clinical Psychology Review, 26*(1), 17–31.

Cahn, B. R., & Polich, J. (2006). Meditation states and traits: EEG, ERP, and neuroimaging studies. *Psychological Bulletin, 132*, 180–211.

Campbell-Sills, L., Barlow, D. H., Brown, T. A., & Hofmann, S. G. (2006). Effects of suppression and acceptance on emotional responses on individuals with anxiety and mood disorders. *Behavior Research and Therapy, 44*, 1251–1263.

Carlson, L. E., & Brown, K. W. (2005). Validation of the Mindful Attention Awareness Scale in a cancer population. *Journal of Psychosomatic Research, 58*, 29–33.

Carlson, L. E., Speca, M., Faris, P., & Patel, K. D. (2007). One year pre–post intervention follow-up of psychological, immune, endocrine and blood pressure outcomes of mindfulness-based stress reduction (MBSR) in breast and prostate cancer outpatients. *Brain, Behavior, and Immunity, 21*(8), 1038–1049.

Carmody, J. (2009). Invited commentary: Evolving conceptions of mindfulness in clinical settings. *Journal of Cognitive Psychotherapy, 23*, 270–280.

Carmody, J., & Baer, R. A. (2008). Relationships between mindfulness practice and levels of mindfulness, medical and psychological symptoms and well-being in a mindfulness-based stress reduction program. *Journal of Behavioral Medicine, 31*(1), 23–33.

Carmody, J., Baer, R. A., Lykins, E. L. B., & Olendzki, N. (2009). An empirical study of the mechanisms of mindfulness in a mindfulness-based stress reduction program. *Journal of Clinical Psychology, 65*(6), 613–626.

Carson, J. W., Carson, K. M., Gil, K. M., & Baucom, D. H. (2004). Mindfulness-based relationship enhancement. *Behavior Therapy, 35*, 471–494.

Cerutti, D. T. (1989). Discrimination theory of rule-governed behavior. *Journal of the Experimental Analysis of Behavior, 51*, 259–276.

Chambers, R., Lo, B. C. Y., & Allen, N. B. (2008). The impact of intensive mindfulness training on attentional control, cognitive style, and affect. *Cognitive Therapy and Research, 32*, 303–322.

Chambless, D. L., & Ollendick, T. H. (2001). Empirically supported psychological interventions: Controversies and evidence. *Annual Review of Psychology, 52*(1), 685–716.

Chan, D., & Woollacott, M. (2007). Effects of level of meditation experience on attentional focus: Is the efficiency of executive or orientation networks improved? *Journal of Alternative and Complementary Medicine, 13*, 651–658.

Chang, V. Y., Palesh, O., Caldwell, R., Glasgow, N., Abramson, M., Luskin, F., et al. (2004). The effects of a mindfulness-based stress reduction program on stress, mindfulness self-efficacy, and positive states of mind. *Stress and Health, 20*(3), 141–147.

Chapman, A. L., Gratz, K. L., & Brown, M. Z. (2006). Solving the puzzle of deliberate self-harm: The experiential avoidance model. *Behaviour Research and Therapy, 44*, 371–394.

Chawla, N., & Ostafin, B. (2007). Experiential avoidance as a functional dimensional approach to psychopathology: An empirical review. *Journal of Clinical Psychology, 63*, 871–890.

Chen, S., & Ravallion, M. (2008). *The developing world is poorer than we thought, but no less successful in the fight against poverty* (World Bank Policy Research Working Paper Series 4703). Washington, DC: Development Research Group, World Bank.

Cheung, M. S. P., Gilbert, P., & Irons, C. (2004). An exploration of shame, social rank, and rumination in relation to depression. *Personality and Individual Differences, 36*, 1143–1153.

Chiesa, A., Calati, R., & Serretti, A. (2011). Does mindfulness training improve cognitive abilities?: A systematic review of neuropsychological findings. *Clinical Psychology Review, 31*, 449–464.

Chiles, J. A., & Strosahl, K. D. (2005). *Clinical manual for assessment and treatment of suicidal patients.* Washington, DC: American Psychiatric Publishing.

Chödrön, P. (2003). *Start where you are: A guide to compassionate living.* Boston: Shambhala.

Chödrön, P. (2007). *No time to lose: A timely guide to the way of the bodhisattva.* Boston: Shambhala.

Chödrön, P. (2012). *Don't believe everything you think: Cultivating a compassionate mind.* Boston: Shambhala.

Clark, D. M., Salkovskis, P. M., Hackmann, A., Wells, A., Ludgate, J., & Gelder, M. (1999). Brief cognitive therapy for panic disorder: A randomized controlled trial. *Journal of Consulting and Clinical Psychology, 67*(4), 583–589.

Clark, H. H. (1996). *Using language* (Vol. 4). Cambridge, UK: Cambridge University Press.

Cleary, T. F. (1994). *Dhammapada: The sayings of Buddha*. New York: Bantam Books.

Cochrane, A., Barnes-Holmes, D., Barnes-Holmes, Y., Stewart, I., & Luciano, C. (2007). Experiential avoidance and aversive visual images: Response delays and event-related potentials on a simple matching task. *Behaviour Research and Therapy, 45*(6), 1379–1388.

Coelho, H. F., Canter, P. H., & Ernst, E. (2007). Mindfulness-based cognitive therapy: evaluating current evidence and informing future research. *Journal of Consulting and Clinical Psychology, 75*(6), 1000–1005.

Coffey, K. A., & Hartman, M. (2008). Mechanisms of action in the inverse relationship between mindfulness and psychological distress. *Complementary Health Practice Review, 13,* 79–91.

Colby F. (1991). An analogue study of the initial carryover effects of meditation, hypnosis, and relaxation using naïve college students. *Biofeedback and Self-Regulation, 16,* 157–165.

Collier, I. D. (2011). *Chinese mythology rocks!* New York: Enslow.

Condon, P., & DeSteno, D. (2011). Compassion for one reduces punishment for another. *Journal of Experimental Social Psychology, 47*(3), 698–701.

Cooper, M. (2012). *The compassionate mind approach to reducing stress: Using compassion focused therapy*. London: Constable & Robinson.

Corcoran, K. M., Farb, N., Anderson, A., & Segal, Z. V. (2010). Mindfulness and emotion regulation: Outcomes and possible mediating mechanisms. In A. M. Kring & D. M. Sloan (Eds.), *Emotion regulation and psychopathology: A transdiagnostic approach to etiology and treatment* (pp. 339–355). New York: Guilford Press.

Corrigan, F. M. (2004). Psychotherapy as assisted homeostasis: Activation of emotional processing mediated by the anterior cingulate cortex. *Medical Hypotheses, 63,* 968–973.

Crane, R. (2009). *Mindfulness-based cognitive therapy*. New York: Routledge.

Craske, M. G., Kircanski, K., Zelikowsky, M., Mystkowski, J., Chowdhury, N., & Baker, A. (2008). Optimizing inhibitory learning during exposure therapy. *Behaviour Research and Therapy, 46,* 5–27.

Cree, M. (2010). Compassion focused therapy with perinatal and mother–infant distress. *International Journal of Cognitive Therapy, 3,* 159–171.

Critchely, H. D. (2005). Neural mechanisms of autonomic, affective and cognitive integration. *Journal of Comparative Neurology, 493,* 154–166.

Crocker, J., & Canevello, A. (2008). Creating and undermining social support in communal relationships: the role of compassionate and self-image goals. *Journal of Personality and Social Psychology, 95*(3), 555–575.

Dahl, J., Lundgren, T., Plumb, J., & Stewart, I. (2009). *The art and science of valuing in psychotherapy: Helping patients discover, explore, and commit to valued action using acceptance and commitment therapy*. Oakland, CA: New Harbinger.

Dalai Lama, H. H. (1991). The Buddhist concept of mind. Mind science: An East–West dialogue. In H. H. Dalai Lama, H. Benson, R. A. F. Thurman, H. E. Gardner, & D. Goleman (Eds.), *Mind science: An East–West dialogue* (pp. 11–18). Somerville, MA: Wisdom.

Dalai Lama, H. H. (1994). *A flash of lightning in the dark of night: A guide to the Bodhisattva's way of life.* Boston: Shambhala.

Dalai Lama, H. H. (2001). *Stages of meditation.* Ithaca, NY: Snow Lion.

Dalai Lama, H. H. (2005a). *Essence of the Heart Sutra: The Dalai Lama's heart of wisdom teachings.* Somerville, MA: Wisdom.

Dalai Lama, H. H. (2005b). *The universe in a single atom.* New York: Morgan Road Books.

Dalai Lama, H. H. (2011). *The transformed mind.* London, UK: Hachette.

Dalai Lama, H. H., & Ekman, P. (2008). *Emotional awareness: Overcoming the obstacles to psychological balance and compassion.* New York: Macmillan.

Damasio, A., & Dolan, R. J. (1999). The feeling of what happens. *Nature, 401,* 847–847.

Das, L. S. (1997). *Awakening the Buddha within.* New York: Broadway.

Davidson, R. J. (2010). Empirical explorations of mindfulness: Conceptual and methodological conundrums. *Emotion, 10*(1), 8–11.

Davidson, R. J., Jackson, D. C., & Kalin, N. H. (2000). Emotion, plasticity, context, and regulation: Perspectives from affective neuroscience. *Psychological Bulletin, 126,* 890–909.

Davidson, R. J., Kabat-Zinn, J., Schumacher, J., Rosenkranz, M., Muller, D., Santorelli, S. F., et al. (2003). Alterations in brain and immune function produced by mindfulness meditation. *Psychosomatic Medicine, 65,* 564–570.

Davis, D. M., & Hayes, J. A. (2011). What are the benefits of mindfulness?: A practice review of psychotherapy-related research. *Psychotherapy, 48*(2), 198–208.

Deikman, A. (1982). *The observing self: Mysticism and psychotherapy.* Boston: Beacon Press.

Dekeyser, M., Raes, F., Leijssen, M. L., Leysen, S. S., & Dewulf, D. (2008). Mindfulness skills and interpersonal behavior. *Personality and Individual Differences, 44,* 1235–1245.

de la Fuente, M., Franco, C., & Salvador, M. (2010). Reduction of blood pressure in a group of hypertensive teachers through a program of mindfulness meditation. *Behavioral Psychology-Psicologia Conductual, 18*(3), 533–552.

DelMonte, M. M. (1995). Meditation and the unconscious. *Journal of Contemporary Psychotherapy, 25*(3), 223–242.

DeRubeis, R. J., Tang, T. Z., & Beck, A. T. (2001). Cognitive therapy. In K. S. Dobson (Ed.), *Handbook of cognitive-behavioral therapies* (2nd ed., pp. 349–392). New York: Guilford Press.

de Silva, P., (2005). *An introduction to Buddhist psychology* (4th ed.). London: Palgrave Macmillan.

Desimone, R., & Duncan, J. (1995). Neural mechanisms of selective visual attention. *Annual Review of Neuroscience, 18*(1), 193–222.

Didonna, F. (2009). *Mindfulness-based interventions in an inpatient setting.* In F. Didonna (Ed.), *Clinical handbook of mindfulness* (pp. 447–462). New York: Springer.

Dimidjian, S., & Linehan, M. M. (2003). Defining an agenda for future research on the clinical application of mindfulness practice. *Clinical Psychology: Science and Practice, 10,* 166–171.

Dobson, K. S. (Ed.). (2009). *Handbook of cognitive-behavioral therapies* (3rd ed.). New York: Guilford Press.

Domjan, M. (1998). *Principles of learning and behavior* (4th ed.). Pacific Grove, CA: Brooks-Cole.

Domjan, M. (2005). Pavlovian conditioning: A functional perspective. *Annual Review of Psychology, 56,* 179–206.

Donohue, B., Tracy, K., & Gorney, S. (2009). Anger (negative impulse) control. In W. T. O'Donohue & J. E. Fisher (Eds.), *General principles and empirically supported techniques of cognitive behavior therapy* (pp. 115–123). Hoboken, NJ: Wiley.

Dowd, T., & McCleery, A. (2007). Elements of Buddhist philosophy in cognitive psychotherapy: The role of cultural specifics and universals. *Journal of Cognitive and Behavioral Psychotherapies, 7,* 67–79.

Dryden, W., & Still, A. (2006). Historical aspects of mindfulness and self-acceptance in psychotherapy. *Journal of Rational–Emotive and Cognitive-Behavior Therapy, 24,* 3–28.

Duncan, J. (1980). The locus of interference in the perception of simultaneous stimuli. *Psychological Review, 87*(3), 272–300.

Dunkley, D. M., Zuroff, D. C., & Blankstein, K. R. (2003). Self-critical perfectionism and daily affect: Dispositional and situational influences on stress and coping. *Journal of Personality and Social Psychology, 84,* 234–252.

Dunkley, D. M., Zuroff, D. C., & Blankstein, K. R. (2006). Specific perfectionism components versus self-criticism in predicting maladjustment. *Personality and Individual Differences, 40,* 665–676.

Dunn, B. R., Hartigan, J. A., & Mikulas, W. L. (1999). Concentration and mindfulness meditations: Unique forms of consciousness? *Applied Psychophysiology and Biofeedback, 24,* 147–165.

Dymond, S., Roche, B., & Bennett, M. (2013). Relational frame theory and experimental psychopathology. In S. Dymond & B. Roche (Eds.), *Advances in relational frame theory and contextual behavioral science: Research and application* (pp. 199–210). Oakland, CA: New Harbinger.

Ekers, D., Richards, D., & Gilbody, S. (2008). A meta-analysis of randomized trials of behavioural treatment of depression. *Psychological Medicine, 38,* 611–624.

Ellis, A. (1962). *Reason and emotion in psychotherapy.* New York: Carol.

Ellis, A. (2006). *The myth of self-esteem: How rational emotive behavior therapy can change your life forever.* New York: Prometheus Books.

Emmons, R. A., & McCullough, M. E. (2003). Counting blessings versus burdens: An experimental investigation of gratitude and subjective well-being in daily life. *Journal of Personality and Social Psychology, 84,* 377–389.

Engström, M., & Söderfeldt, B. (2010). Brain activation during compassion meditation: A case study. *Journal of Alternative and Complementary Medicine, 16*(5), 597–599.

Epstein, N. (1995). *Thoughts without a thinker*. New York: Basic Books.

Farb, N. A. S., Anderson, A. K., Mayberg, H., Bean, J., McKeon, D., & Segal, Z. V. (2010). Minding one's emotions: Mindfulness training alters the neural expression of sadness. *Emotion, 10*, 25–33.

Farb, N. A. S., Segal, Z., Mayberg, V., Bean, H. J., McKeon, D., Fatima, Z., et al. (2007). Attending to the present: Mindfulness meditation reveals distinct neural modes of self-reference. *Social Cognitive and Affective Neuroscience, 2*(4), 313–322.

Festinger, L. (1957). *A theory of cognitive dissonance*. Stanford, CA: Stanford University Press.

Fledderus, M., Bohlmeijer, E. T., Smit, F., & Westerhof, G. J. (2010). Mental health promotion as a new goal in public mental health care: A randomized controlled trial of an intervention enhancing psychological flexibility. *American Journal of Public Health, 100*(12), 2372.

Fletcher, L. B., Schoendorff, B., & Hayes, S. C. (2010). Searching for mindfulness in the brain: A process-oriented approach to examining the neural correlates of mindfulness. *Mindfulness, 1*, 41–63.

Follette, V. M., Palm, K. M., & Hall, M. L. R. (2004). Acceptance, mindfulness, and trauma. In S. C. Hayes, V. M. Follette, M. Victoria, & M. M. Linehan (Eds.), *Mindfulness and acceptance: Expanding the cognitive-behavioral tradition* (pp. 192–208). New York: Guilford Press.

Forrest, M. S., & Hokanson, J. E. (1975). Depression and autonomic arousal reduction accompanying self-punitive behavior. *Journal of Abnormal Psychology, 84*(4), 346.

Forsyth, J. P., & Eifert, G. H. (2007). *The mindfulness and acceptance workbook for anxiety*. Oakland, CA: New Harbinger.

Forsyth, J. P., Parker, J. D., & Finlay, C. G. (2003). Anxiety sensitivity, controllability, and experiential avoidance and their relation to drug of choice and addiction severity in a residential sample of substance-abusing veterans. *Addictive Behaviors, 28*(5), 851–870.

Fredrickson, B. L., & Branigan, C. (2005). Positive emotions broaden the scope of attention and thought–action repertoires. *Cognition and Emotion, 19*, 313–332.

Fredrickson, B. L., Cohn, M. A., Coffey, K. A., Pek, J., & Finkel, S. M. (2008). Open hearts build lives: Positive emotions, induced through loving-kindness meditation, build consequential personal resources. *Journal of Personality and Social Psychology, 95*(5), 1045.

Frewen, P. A., Evans, E. M., Maraj, N., Dozois, D. J. A., & Partridge, K. (2008). Letting go: Mindfulness and negative automatic thinking. *Cognitive Therapy Research, 32*, 758–774.

Friedlander, P. G. (2009). Dhammapada traditions and translations. *Journal of Religious History, 33*, 215–234.

Fulton, P. R., & Seigel, R. D. (2005). Buddhist and Western psychology: Seeking common ground. In C. K. Germer, R. D. Siegel & P. R. Fulton (Eds.), *Mindfulness and psychotherapy* (pp. 36 –58). New York: Guilford Press.

Gale, C., Gilbert, P., Read, N., & Goss, K. (2014). An evaluation of the impact of introducing compassion focused therapy to a standard treatment programme for people with eating disorders. *Clinical Psychology and Psychotherapy, 21*(1), 1–12.

Germer, C. K. (2005a). Mindfulness: What is it? Does it matter? In C. K. Germer, R. D. Seigel, & P. R. Fulton (Eds.), *Mindfulness and psychotherapy* (pp. 3–27). New York: Guilford Press.

Germer, C. K. (2005b). Teaching mindfulness in therapy. In C. K. Germer, R. D. Seigel, & P. R. Fulton (Eds.), *Mindfulness and psychotherapy* (pp. 113–129). New York: Guilford Press.

Germer, C. K. (2009). *The mindful path to self-compassion: Freeing yourself from destructive thoughts and emotions.* New York: Guilford Press.

Germer, C. K. (2013). Cultivating compassion in psychotherapy. In C. K. Germer & R. D. Siegel (Eds.), *Wisdom and compassion in psychotherapy: Deepening mindfulness in clinical practice* (pp. 93–110). New York: Guilford Press.

Germer, C. K., & Neff, K. D. (2011, July 21). *Mindful self-compassion training (MSC).* Paper presented at the Max Planck Institute for Human and Cognitive Brain Sciences conference "How to Train Compassion," Berlin, Germany.

Germer, C. K., Siegel, R. D., & Fulton, P. R. (Eds.). (2005). *Mindfulness and psychotherapy.* New York: Guilford Press.

Gifford, E. V., Kohlenberg, B. S., Hayes, S. C., Antonuccio, D. O., Piasecki, M. M., & Rasmussen-Gilbert, P. (1989). *Human nature and suffering.* London: Erlbaum.

Gilbert, P. (1998a). The evolved basis and adaptive functions of cognitive distortions. *British Journal of Medical Psychology, 71*, 447–64.

Gilbert, P. (1998b). What is shame?: Some core issues and controversies. In P. Gilbert & B. Andrews (Eds.), *Shame: Interpersonal behavior, psychopathology, and culture* (pp. 3–38). New York: Oxford University Press.

Gilbert, P. (2001). Evolutionary approaches to psychopathology: The role of natural defenses. *Australian and New Zealand Journal of Psychiatry, 35*, 17–27.

Gilbert, P. (Ed.). (2005a). *Compassion: Conceptualizations, research and use in psychotherapy.* New York: Routledge.

Gilbert, P. (2005b). Compassion and cruelty. In P. Gilbert (Ed.), *Compassion: Conceptualizations, research, and use in psychotherapy* (pp. 9–74). New York: Routledge.

Gilbert, P. (2007). Evolved minds and compassion in the therapeutic relationship. In P. Gilbert & R. Leahy (Eds.), *The therapeutic relationship in the cognitive behavioral psychotherapies* (pp. 106–142). New York: Routledge.

Gilbert, P. (2009a). *The compassionate mind.* London: Constable & Robinson.

Gilbert, P. (2009b). Introducing compassion-focused therapy. *Advances in Psychiatric Treatment, 15*, 199–209.

Gilbert, P. (2009c). *Overcoming depression: A guide to recovery* (rev. 3rd ed.). London: Constable & Robinson.

Gilbert, P. (2010a). *Compassion-focused therapy.* London: Routledge.

Gilbert, P. (2010b). Compassion focused therapy: A special section. *International Journal of Cognitive Therapy, 3*(2), 95–96.

Gilbert, P. (2010c). An introduction to compassion focused therapy in cognitive behavior therapy. *International Journal of Cognitive Therapy, 3*, 97–112.

Gilbert, P., Baldwin, M. W., Irons, C., Baccus, J. R., & Palmer, M. (2006). Self-criticism and self-warmth: An imagery study exploring their relation to depression. *Journal of Cognitive Psychotherapy, 20*(2), 183–200.

Gilbert, P., & Irons, C. (2005). Focused therapies and compassionate mind training for shame and self-attacking. In P. Gilbert (Ed.), *Compassion: Conceptualizations, research and use in psychotherapy* (pp. 263–326). New York: Routledge.

Gilbert, P., & Leahy, R. (2007). *The therapeutic relationship in the cognitive behavioral psychotherapies.* New York: Routledge.

Gilbert, P., McEwan, K., Irons, C., Bhundia, R., Christie, R., Broomhead, C., et al. (2010). Self-harm in a mixed clinical population: The roles of self-criticism, shame, and social rank. *British Journal of Clinical Psychology, 49*, 563–576.

Gilbert, P., & Procter, S. (2006). Compassionate mind training for people with high shame and self-criticism: Overview and pilot study of a group. *Clinical Psychology and Psychotherapy, 13*, 353–379.

Gilbert, P., & Waltz, J. (2010). Mindfulness and health behaviors. *Mindfulness, 1*, 227–234.

Goldstein, J., & Kornfield, J. (1987). *Seeking the heart of wisdom.* Boston: Shambhala.

Goleman, D. (1988). *The meditative mind.* New York: Putnam.

Goleman, D. (1991). A Western perspective. In D. P. Goleman & R. A. Thurman (Eds.), *Mind–science: An East–West dialogue* (pp. 3–7). Somerville, MA: Wisdom.

Goodman, T. A. (2005). Working with children: Beginner's mind. In C. K. Germer, R. D. Seigel, & P. R. Fulton (Eds.), *Mindfulness and psychotherapy* (pp. 197–219). New York: Guilford Press.

Goss, K. (2011). *The compassionate mind approach to beating overeating: Using compassion-focused therapy.* London: Constable & Robinson.

Goss, K., & Allen, S. (2010). Compassion focused therapy for eating disorders. *International Journal of Cognitive Therapy, 3*, 141–158.

Gottman, J. M. (1999). *The marriage clinic: A scientifically-based marital therapy.* New York: Norton.

Greene, B. (1999). *The elegant universe.* New York: Norton.

Greeson, J. M. (2009). Mindfulness research update: 2008. *Complementary Health Practice Review, 14*(1), 10–18.

Greeson, J., & Brantley, J. (2009). Mindfulness and anxiety disorders: Developing a wise relationship with the inner experience of fear. In F. Didonna (Ed.), *Clinical handbook of mindfulness* (pp. 171–188). New York: Springer.

Gross, J. J., & John, O. P. (2003). Individual differences in two emotion regulation processes: Implications for affect, relationships, and well-being. *Journal of Personality and Social Psychology, 85*, 348–362.

Grossman, P., Neimann, L., Schmidt, S., & Walach, H. (2004). Mindfulness-based stress reduction and health benefits: A meta-analysis. *Journal of Psychosomatic Research, 57*, 35–43.

Guenther, H. V, & Kawamura, L. S. (1975). *Mind in Buddhist psychology.* Berkeley, CA: Dharma.

Gunaratana, B. H. (2002). *Mindfulness in plain English.* Somerville, MA: Wisdom.

Hale, L., Strauss, C., & Taylor, B. L. (2013). The effectiveness and acceptability of mindfulness-based therapy for obsessive compulsive disorder: A review of the literature. *Mindfulness, 4*(4), 375–382.

Hamilton, N. A., Kitzman, H., & Gutotte, S. (2006). Enhancing health and emotion: Mindfulness as a missing link between cognitive therapy and positive psychology. *Journal of Cognitive Psychotherapy, 20,* 123–134.

Hannan, S. E., & Tolin, D. F. (2005). Mindfulness- and acceptance-based behavior therapy for obsessive-compulsive disorder. In S. M. Orsillo & L. Roemer (Eds.), *Acceptance and mindfulness-based approaches to anxiety* (pp. 271–299). New York: Springer.

Hartnett, S. J. (2010). Communication, social justice, and joyful commitment. *Western Journal of Communication, 74,* 68–93.

Hawton, K. E., Salkovskis, P. M., Kirk, J. E., & Clark, D. M. (1989). *Cognitive behaviour therapy for psychiatric problems: A practical guide.* Oxford, UK: Oxford University Press.

Hayes, A. M., & Feldman, G. (2004). Clarifying the construct of mindfulness in the context of emotion regulation and the process of change in therapy. *Clinical Psychology: Science and Practice, 11,* 255–262.

Hayes, S. C. (2002a). Acceptance, mindfulness and science. *Clinical Psychology Science and Practice, 9,* 101–106.

Hayes, S. C. (2002b). Buddhism and acceptance and commitment therapy. *Cognitive and Behavioral Practice, 9,* 58–66.

Hayes, S. C. (2004a). Acceptance and commitment therapy and the new behavior therapies. In S. C. Hayes, V. M. Follette, & M. M. Linehan (Eds.), *Mindfulness and acceptance* (pp. 1–29). New York: Guilford Press.

Hayes, S. C. (2004b). Acceptance and commitment therapy, relational frame theory, and the third wave of behavioral and cognitive therapies. *Behavior Therapy, 35*(4), 639–665.

Hayes, S. C. (2008a). Avoiding the mistakes of the past. *Behavior Therapist, 31*(8), 150.

Hayes, S. C. (2008b). Climbing our hills: A beginning conversation on the comparison of acceptance and commitment therapy and traditional cognitive behavioral therapy. *Clinical Psychology: Science and Practice, 15*(4), 286–295.

Hayes, S. C., Follette, V. M., & Linehan, M. M. (Eds.). (2004). *Mindfulness and acceptance: Expanding the cognitive-behavioral tradition.* New York: Guilford Press.

Hayes, S. C., Luoma, J., Bond, F., Masuda, A., & Lillis, J. (2006). Acceptance and commitment therapy: Model, processes, and outcomes. *Behaviour Research and Therapy, 44*(1), 1–25.

Hayes, S. C., Orsillo, S. M., & Roemer, L. (2010). Changes in proposed mechanisms of action during an acceptance based behavior therapy for generalized anxiety disorder. *Behaviour Research and Therapy, 48*(3), 238–245.

Hayes, S. C., & Shenk, C. (2004). Operationalizing mindfulness without unnecessary attachments. *Clinical Psychology Science and Practice, 11,* 249–254.

Hayes, S. C., & Smith, S. (2005). *Get out of your mind and into your life: The new acceptance and commitment therapy.* Oakland, CA: New Harbinger.

Hayes, S. C., Stroshal, K. D., & Wilson, K. G. (1999). *Acceptance and commitment therapy: An experiential approach to behavior change.* New York: Guilford Press.

Hayes, S. C., Strosahl, K. D., & Wilson, K. G. (2011). *Acceptance and commitment therapy: The process and practice of mindful change* (2nd ed.). New York: Guilford Press.

Hayes, S. C., Strosahl, K. D., Wilson, K. G., Bissett, R. T., Pistorello, J., Toarmino, D., et al. (2004). Measuring experiential avoidance: A preliminary test of a working model. *Psychological Record, 54,* 553–578.

Hayes, S. C., Villatte, M., Levin, M., & Hildebrandt, M. (2011). Open, aware, and active: Contextual approaches as an emerging trend in the behavioral and cognitive therapies. *Annual Review of Clinical Psychology, 7,* 141–168.

Hayes, S. C., & Wilson, K. G. (2003). Mindfulness: Method and process. *Clinical Psychology, 10,* 161–165.

Hayes, S. C., Wilson, K. G., Gifford, E. V., Follette, V. M., & Strosahl, K. D. (1996). Experiential avoidance and behavioral disorders: A functional dimensional approach to diagnosis and treatment. *Journal of Consulting and Clinical Psychology, 64,* 1152–1168.

Hayes, S. C., Zettle, R. D., & Rosenfarb, I. (1989). Rule following. In S. C. Hayes (Ed.), *Rule-governed behavior: Cognition, contingencies, and instructional control* (pp. 191–220). New York: Plenum Press.

Hayes, S. K. (1992). *Enlightened self-protection: The kasumi-an ninja art tradition: An original workbook.* Dayton, OH: Nine Gates Press.

Heeren, A., Van Broeck, N., & Philippot, P. (2009). The effects of mindfulness on executive processes and autobiographical memory specificity. *Behaviour Research and Therapy, 48,* 403–409.

Henderson, L. (2010). *Improving social confidence and reducing shyness: Using compassion focused therapy.* London: Constable & Robinson.

Herbert, J. D., & Forman, E. M. (2011). The evolution of cognitive behavior therapy: The rise of psychological acceptance and mindfulness. In J. D. Herbert & E. M. Forman (Eds.), *Acceptance and mindfulness in cognitive behavior therapy: Understanding and applying the new therapies* (pp. 3–25). Hoboken, NJ: Wiley.

Hirst, I. S. (2003). Perspectives on mindfulness. *Journal of Psychiatric and Mental Health Nursing, 1,* 359–366.

Hodgins, H. S., & Adair, K. C. (2010). Attentional processes and meditation. *Consciousness and Cognition, 19,* 872–878.

Hofmann, S. G. (2012). *An introduction to modern CBT: Psychological solutions to mental health problems.* Chichester, UK: Wiley-Blackwell.

Hofmann, S. G., Grossman, P., & Hinton, D. E. (2011). Loving-kindness and compassion meditation: Potential for psychological interventions. *Clinical Psychology Review, 31,* 1126–1132.

Hofmann, S. G., Sawyer, A. T., Witt, A. A., & Oh, D. (2010). The effect of mindfulness-based therapy on anxiety and depression: A meta-analytic review. *Journal of Consulting and Clinical Psychology, 78,* 169–183.

Hölzel, B. K., Carmody, J., Vangel, M., Congleton, C., Yerramsetti, S. M., Gard, T., et al. (2011). Mindfulness practice leads to increases in regional brain gray matter density. *Psychiatry Research: Neuroimaging, 191,* 36–43.

Hölzel, B. K., Lazar, S. W., Gard, T., Schuman-Olivier, Z., Vago, D. R., & Ott, U. (2011). How does mindfulness meditation work?: Proposing mechanisms of action from a conceptual and neural perspective. *Perspectives on Psychological Science, 6*(6), 537–559.

Hölzel, B. K., Ott, U., Gard, T., Hempel, H., Weygandt, M., Morgen, K., et al. (2008). Investigation of mindfulness meditation practitioners with voxel-based morphometry. *Social Cognitive and Affective Neuroscience, 3,* 55–61.

Hutcherson, C. A., Seppala, E. M., & Gross, J. J. (2008). Loving-kindness meditation increases social connectedness. *Emotion, 8*(5), 720–724.

Huston, D. C., Garland, E. L., & Farb, N. A. (2011). Mechanisms of mindfulness in communication training. *Journal of Applied Communication Research, 39,* 406–421.

Irving, L. M., Snyder, C. R., Cheavens, J., Gravel, L., Hanke, J., Hilberg, P., et al. (2004). The relationship between hope and outcomes at the pretreatment, beginning, and later phases of psychotherapy. *Journal of Psychotherapy Integration, 4,* 419–443.

Jacobson, N. S., Dobson, K. S., Truax, P. A., Addis, M. E., Koerner, K., Gollan, J. K., et al. (1996). A component analysis of cognitive-behavioral treatment for depression. *Journal of Consulting and Clinical Psychology, 64,* 295–304.

Jacobson, N. S., Martell, C. R., & Dimidjian, S. (2001). Behavioral activation treatment for depression: Returning to contextual roots. *Clinical Psychology: Science and Practice, 8*(3), 255–270.

James, W. (2009). *The varieties of religious experience.* New York: Createspace. (Original work published 1902)

Jha, A. P., Krompinger, J., & Baime, M. J. (2007). Mindfulness training modifies subsystems of attention. *Cognitive, Affective, and Behavioral Neuroscience, 7*(2), 109–119.

Johnson, D. P., Penn, D. L., Fredrickson, B. L., Meyer, P. S., Kring, A. M., & Brantley, M. (2009). Loving-kindness meditation to enhance recovery from negative symptoms of schizophrenia. *Journal of Clinical Psychology, 65*(5), 499–509.

Josefsson, T., & Broberg, A. (2010). Meditators and non-meditators on sustained and executive attentional performance. *Mental Health, Religion, and Culture, 1,* 1–19.

Judge, L., Cleghorn, A., McEwan, K., & Gilbert, P. (2012). An exploration of group-based compassion focused therapy for a heterogeneous range of clients presenting to a community mental health team. *International Journal of Cognitive Therapy, 5*(4), 420–429.

Kabat-Zinn, J. (1982). An outpatient program in behavioral medicine for chronic pain patients based on the practice of mindfulness meditation:

Theoretical considerations and preliminary results. *General Hospital Psychiatry, 4*(1), 33–47.

Kabat-Zinn, J. (1990). *Full catastrophe living: Using the wisdom of our body and mind to face stress, pain, and illness.* New York: Delta.

Kabat-Zinn, J. (2003). Mindfulness-based interventions in context: Past, present, and future. *Clinical Psychology, 10,* 144–156.

Kabat-Zinn, J. (2005). *Coming to our senses: Healing ourselves and the world through mindfulness.* New York: Hyperion.

Kabat-Zinn, J. (2009). Foreword. In F. Didonna (Ed.), *Clinical handbook of mindfulness* (pp. xxv–xxxiii). New York: Springer.

Kabat-Zinn, J., Massion, A. O., Kristeller, J., Peterson, L. G., Fletcher, K. E., Pbert, L., et al. (1992). Effectiveness of meditation-based stress reduction programs in the treatment of anxiety disorders. *American Journal of Psychiatry, 149,* 936–943.

Kalupahana. (1986). *The philosophy of the Middle Way.* Albany: State University of New York Press.

Kang, C. (2009). Buddhist and tantric perspectives on causality and society. *Journal of Buddhist Ethics, 16,* 69–103.

Kang, C., & Whittingham, K. (2010). Mindfulness: A dialogue between Buddism and clinical psychology. *Mindfulness, 1,* 161–173.

Kanov, J. M., Maitlis, S., Worline, M. C., Dutton, J. E., Frost, P. J., & Lilius, J. M. (2004). Compassion in organizational life. *American Behavioral Scientist, 47*(6), 808–827.

Kasamatsu, A., & Hirai, T. (1973). An electroencephalographic study on Zen mediation (Zazen). *Journal of the American Institute for Hypnosis, 14,* 107–114.

Kashdan, T. B., Breen, W. E., & Julian, T. (2010). Everyday strivings in war veterans with posttraumatic stress disorder: Suffering from a hyper-focus on avoidance and emotion regulation. *Behavior Therapy, 41*(3), 350–363.

Kashdan, T. B., & McKnight, P. E. (2013). Commitment to a purpose in life: An antidote to the suffering by individuals with social anxiety disorder. *Emotion, 13*(6), 1150–1159.

Kazdin, A. E. (1979). Nonspecific treatment factors in psychotherapy outcome research. *Journal of Consulting and Clinical Psychology, 47,* 846–851.

Kelly, A. C., Zuroff, D. C., Foa, C. L., & Gilbert, P. (2010). Who benefits from training in self-compassionate self-regulation?: A study of smoking reduction. *Journal of Social and Clinical Psychology, 29*(7), 727–755.

Kelly, A. C., Zuroff, D. C., & Shapira, L. B. (2009). Soothing oneself and resisting self-attacks: The treatment of two intrapersonal deficits in depression vulnerability. *Cognitive Therapy and Research, 33*(3), 301–313.

Keng, S. L., Smoski, M. J., & Robins, C. J. (2011). Effects of mindfulness on psychological health: A review of empirical studies. *Clinical Psychology Review, 31*(6), 1041–1056.

Kessler, R. C., Chiu, W. T., Demler, O., & Walters, E. E. (2005). Prevalence, severity, and comorbidity of twelve-month DSM-IV disorders in the National Comorbidity Survey Replication (NCS-R). *Archives of General Psychiatry, 62,* 617–627.

Kessler, R. C., McGonagle, K. A., Zhao, S., Nelson, C. B., Hughes, M., Eshleman, S., et al. (1994). Lifetime and 12-month prevalence of DSM-III-R psychiatric disorders in the United States: Results from the National Comorbidity Survey. *Archives of General Psychiatry, 51,* 8–19.

Kim, J., Kim, S., Kim, J., Joeng, B., Park, C., Son, A., et al. (2011). Compassionate attitude towards others' suffering activates the mesolimbic neural system. *Neuropsychologia, 47,* 2073–2081.

Kimbrough, E., Magyari, T., Langenberg, P., Chesney, M., & Berman, B. (2010). Mindfulness intervention for child abuse survivors. *Journal of Clinical Psychology, 66*(1), 17–33.

Kohlenberg, R. J., & Tsai, M. (1991). *Functional analytic psychotherapy.* New York: Springer:

Kolts, R. L. (2012). *The compassionate mind approach to working with your anger: Using compassion-focused therapy.* London: Constable & Robinson.

Kornfield. J. (1993). *A path with heart.* New York: Bantam Books.

Kornfield, J. (2008). *The wise heart.* New York: Bantam Books.

Kosslyn, S. M., Ganis, G., & Thompson, W. L. (2001). Neural foundations of imagery. *Nature Reviews Neuroscience, 2*(9), 635–642.

Krisanaprakornkit, T., Krisanaprakornkit, W., Piyavhatkul, N., & Laopaiboon, M. (2005). Meditation therapy for anxiety disorders. *Cochrane Database of Systematic Reviews,* Issue 1 (Article No. CD004998).

Kurzban, R., & Leary, M. R. (2001). Evolutionary origins of stigmatization: The functions of social exclusion. *Psychological Bulletin, 127*(2), 187–208.

Kuyken, W., Watkins, E., Holden, E., White, K., Taylor, R. S., Byford, S., et al. (2010). How does mindfulness-based cognitive therapy work? *Behaviour Research and Therapy, 48*(11), 1105–1112.

Kwee, M. G. T. (Ed.). (1990). *Psychotherapy, meditation, and health: A cognitive behavioural perspective.* London: East–West.

Kwee, M. G. T. (1998). Relational Buddhism: A psychological quest for meaning and sustainable happiness. In P. T. Wong & P. S. Fry (Eds.), *The human quest for meaning.* (pp. 443–448). Mahwah, NJ: Erlbaum.

Kwee, M. G. T. (2011). Relational Buddhism: An integrative psychology of happiness amidst existential suffering. In I. Boniwell & S. Davis (Eds.), *Oxford handbook of happiness* (pp. 357–370). Oxford, UK: Oxford University Press.

Kwee, M. G. T., & Ellis, A. (1998). The interface between rational emotive behavior therapy (REBT) and Zen. *Journal of rational-emotive and cognitive-behavior therapy, 16,* 5–43.

Kwee, M. G. T., Gergen, K. L., & Koshikawa, F. (2006). *Horizons in Buddhist psychology: Practice, research and theory.* Chagrin Falls, OH: Taos Institute Publications.

Laird, R. S., & Metalsky, G. I. (2009). Attribution change. In W. T. O'Donohue & J. E. Fisher (Eds.), *General principles and empirically supported techniques of cognitive behavior therapy* (pp. 133–137). Hoboken, NJ: Wiley.

Laithwaite, H., O'Hanlon, M., Collins, P., Doyle, P., Abraham, L., Porter, S., et al. (2009). Recovery after psychosis (RAP): A compassion focused programme for individuals residing in high security settings. *Behavioural and Cognitive Psychotherapy, 39,* 511–526.

Lakey, C. E., Campbell, W. K., Brown, K. W., & Goodie, A. S. (2007). Dispositional mindfulness as a predictor of the severity of gambling outcomes. *Personality and Individual Differences, 43*(7), 1698–1710.

Lakey, C. E., Kernis, M. H., Heppner, W. L., & Lance, C. E. (2008). Individual differences in authenticity and mindfulness as predictors of verbal defensiveness. *Journal of Research in Personality, 42*(1), 230–238.

Lazar, S. W., Bush, G., Gollub, R. L., Fricchione, G. L., Khalsa, G., & Benson, H. (2000). Functional brain mapping of the relaxation response and meditation. *NeuroReport, 11,* 1581–1585.

Lazar, S. W., Kerr, C. E., Wasserman, R. H., Gray, J. R., Greve, D. N., Treadway, M. T., et. al. (2005). Meditation experience is associated with increased cortical thickness. *NeuroReport, 16,* 1893–1897.

Leahy, R. L., & Rego, S. (2012). Cognitive restructuring. In W. T. O'Donohue & E. F. Jane (Eds.), *Cognitive behavior therapy: Core principles for practice* (pp. 133–153). Hoboken, NJ: Wiley.

Leahy, R. L., Tirch, D. D., & Napolitano, L. A. (2011). *Emotion regulation in psychotherapy: A practitioner's guide.* New York: Guilford Press.

LeDoux, J. E. (1996). *The emotional brain.* New York: Simon & Schuster.

LeDoux, J. E. (1998). Fear and the brain: Where have we been, and where are we going? *Biological Psychiatry, 44,* 1229–1238.

Ledoux, J. E. (2002). *The synaptic self.* New York: Viking Press.

Lee, D., & James, S. (2012). *The compassionate mind approach to recovering from trauma: Using compassion focused therapy.* London: Constable & Robinson.

Levesque, C., & Brown, K. W. (2007). Mindfulness as a moderator of the effect of implicit motivational self-concept on day-to-day behavioral motivation. *Motivation and Emotion, 31,* 284–299.

Levine, S. (1979). *A gradual awakening.* New York: Anchor Books.

Lieberman, M. D., Eisenberger, N. I., Crockett, M. J., Tom, S. M., Pfeifer, J. H., & Way, B. M. (2007). Putting feelings into words affect labeling disrupts amygdala activity in response to affective stimuli. *Psychological Science, 18,* 421–428.

Lillis, J., & Hayes, S. C. (2007). Applying acceptance, mindfulness, and values to the reduction of prejudice: A pilot study. *Behavior Modification, 31*(4), 389–411.

Lim, S., & Kim, L. (2005). Cognitive processing of emotional information in depression, panic, and somatoform disorder. *Journal of Abnormal Psychology, 114,* 50–61.

Linehan, M. M. (1993a). *Cognitive-behavioral treatment of borderline personality disorder.* New York: Guilford Press.

Linehan, M. M. (1993b). *Skills training manual for treating borderline personality disorder.* New York: Guilford Press.

Longe, O., Maratos, F. A., Gilbert, P., Evans, G., Volker, F., Rockliff, H., et al. (2010). Having a word with yourself: Neural correlates of self-criticism and self-reassurance. *NeuroImage, 49,* 1849–1856.

Lopez Jr., D. S. (2009). *Buddhism and science: A guide for the perplexed*. Chicago: University of Chicago Press.

Lovibond, P. F., Mitchell, C. J., Minard, E., Brady, A., & Menzies, R. G. (2009). Safety behaviours preserve threat beliefs: Protection from extinction of human fear conditioning by an avoidance response. *Behaviour Research and Therapy, 47*, 716–720.

Lucre, K. M., & Corten, N. (2013). An exploration of group compassion-focused therapy for personality disorder. *Psychology and Psychotherapy: Theory, Research and Practice, 85*, 387–400.

Lutz, A., Brefczynski-Lewis, J., Johnstone, T., & Davidson, R. J. (2008). Regulation of the neural circuitry of emotion by compassion meditation: Effects of meditative expertise. *PLoS ONE, 3*, 1–10.

Lutz, A., Greischar, L. L., Rawlings, N. B., Ricard, M., & Davidson, R. J. (2004). Long-term meditators self-induce high-amplitude gamma synchrony during mental practice. *Proceedings of the National Academy of Sciences of the United States of America, 101*(46), 16369–16373.

Lutz, A., Slagter, H. A., Dunne, J. D., & Davidson, R. J. (2008). Attention regulation and monitoring in meditation. *Trends in Cognitive Sciences, 12*(4), 163–169

Lutz, A., Slagter, H. A., Rawlings, N. B., Francis, A. D., Greischar, L. L., & Davidson, R. J. (2009). Mental training enhances attentional stability: Neural and behavioral evidence. *Journal of Neuroscience, 29*, 13418–13427.

Makransky, J. (2012). Compassion in Buddhist psychology. In C. K. Germer & R. D. Siegel (Eds.), *Compassion and wisdom in psychotherapy* (pp. 61–74). New York: Guilford Press.

Mansell, W. (2008). What is CBT really and how can we enhance the impact of effective psychotherapies such as CBT? In R. House & D. Loewenthal (Eds.), *Against and for CBT: Towards a constructive dialogue* (pp. 19–32). Herefordshire, UK: PCCS Books.

Marlatt, G. A., & Donovan, D. M. (Eds.). (2005). *Relapse prevention: Maintenance strategies in the treatment of addictive behaviors*. New York: Guilford Press.

Marshall, M. B., Zuroff, D. C., McBride, C., & Bagby, R. M. (2008). Self-criticism predicts differential response to treatment for major depression. *Journal of Clinical Psychology, 64*(3), 231–244.

Martell, C. R., Addis, M. E., & Jacobson, N. S. (2001). *Depression in context: Strategies for guided action*. New York: Norton.

Martin, J. R. (1997). Mindfulness: A proposed common factor. *Journal of Psychotherapy Integration, 7*, 291–312.

Marx, B. P., & Sloan, D. M. (2005). Peritraumatic dissociation and experiential avoidance as predictors of posttraumatic stress symptomatology. *Behaviour Research and Therapy, 43*(5), 569–583.

Mayhew, S. L., & Gilbert, P. (2008). Compassionate mind training with people who hear malevolent voices: A case series report. *Clinical Psychology and Psychotherapy, 15*, 113–138.

McDonald, K., & Courtin, R. (2005). *How to meditate: A practical guide* (2nd ed.). Somerville, MA: Wisdom.

McDowd, J. M. (2007). An overview of attention: Behavior and brain. *Journal of Neurologic Physical Therapy, 31*(3), 98–103.

Miller, J. J., Fletcher, K., & Kabat-Zinn, J. (1995). Three-year follow-up and clinical implications of a mindfulness meditation-based stress reduction intervention in the treatment of anxiety disorders. *General Hospital Psychiatry, 17,* 192–200.

Mingyur, R. Y. (2007). *The joy of living: Unlocking the secret and science of happiness.* New York: Harmony Books.

Mingyur, R. Y., Rinpoche, Y. M., & Swanson, E. (2010). *Joyful wisdom.* New York: Random House.

Mirsky, A. F., Anthony, B. J., Duncan, C. C., Ahearn, M. B., & Kellam, S. G. (1991). Analysis of the elements of attention: A neuropsychological approach. *Neuropsychology Review, 2,* 109–145.

Mogg, K., Bradley, B. P., Williams, R., & Mathews, A. (1993). Subliminal processing of emotional information in anxiety and depression. *Journal of Abnormal Psychology, 102,* 304–311.

Moore, A., & Malinowski, P. (2009). Meditation, mindfulness and cognitive flexibility. *Consciousness and Cognition, 18*(1), 176–186.

Mosig, Y. D. (1989). Wisdom and compassion: What the Buddha taught a psycho-poetical analysis. *Journal of Theoretical and Philosophical Psychology, 9,* 27–36.

Moyers, B. (1993). *Healing the mind.* New York: Doubleday.

Neely, M. E., Schallert, D. L., Mohammed, S. S., Roberts, R. M., & Chen, Y. (2009). Self-kindness when facing stress: The role of self-compassion, goal regulation, and support in college students' well-being. *Motivation and Emotion, 33,* 88–97.

Neff, K. D. (2003a). The development and validation of a scale to measure self-compassion. *Self and Identity, 2,* 223–250.

Neff, K. D. (2003b). Self-compassion: An alternative conceptualization of a healthy attitude toward oneself. *Self and Identity, 2,* 85–101.

Neff, K. D. (2009). The role of self-compassion in development: A healthier way to relate to oneself. *Human Development, 52,* 211–214.

Neff, K. D. (2011a). Self-compassion, self-esteem, and well-being. *Social and Personality Psychology Compass, 5,* 1–12.

Neff, K. (2011b). *Self-compassion: The proven power of being kind to yourself.* New York: HarperCollins.

Neff, K. D. (2012). The science of self-compassion. In C. Germer & R. Siegel (Eds.), *Compassion and wisdom in psychotherapy* (pp. 79–92). New York: Guilford Press.

Neff, K. D., & Germer, C. K. (2011, July). *Mindful self-compassion training.* Presented at the Max Planck Institute, Berlin, Germany.

Neff, K. D., & Germer, C. K. (2013). A pilot study and randomized controlled trial of the mindful self-compassion program. *Journal of Clinical Psychology, 69*(1), 28–44.

Neff, K. D., Hseih, Y., & Dejithirat, K. (2005). Self-compassion, achievement goals, and coping with academic failure. *Self and Identity, 4,* 263–287.

Neff, K. D., Kirkpatrick, K., & Rude, S. S. (2007). Self-compassion and its link to adaptive psychological functioning. *Journal of Research in Personality,* *41,* 139–154.

Neff, K. D., Pisitsungkagarn, K., & Hseih, Y. (2008). Self-compassion and self-construal in the United States, Thailand, and Taiwan. *Journal of Cross-Cultural Psychology, 39,* 267–285.

Neff, K. D., Rude, S. S., & Kirkpatrick, K. (2007). An examination of self-compassion in relation to positive psychological functioning and personality traits. *Journal of Research in Personality, 41,* 908–916.

Neff, K. D., & Vonk, R. (2009). Self-compassion versus global self-esteem: Two different ways of relating to oneself. *Journal of Personality, 77,* 23–50.

Nhat Hanh, T. (1973). *The heart of Buddhist teachings.* Boston: Shambhala.

Nhat Hanh, T. (1975). *The miracles of mindfulness: A manual on meditation.* Boston: Beacon Press.

Nhat Hanh, T. (1998). *The heart of the Buddha's teaching.* Berkeley, CA: Parallax Press.

Nolen-Hoeksema, S. (2000). The role of rumination in depressive disorders and mixed anxiety/depressive symptoms. *Journal of Abnormal Psychology, 109,* 504–511.

Nyanaponika, T. (1973). *The heart of Buddhist meditation.* New York: Weiser Books.

Olendzki, A. (2005). The roots of mindfulness. In C. K. Germer, R. D. Seigel, & P. R. Fulton (Eds.), *Mindfulness and psychotherapy* (pp. 241–261). New York: Guilford Press.

Olendzki, A. (2010). *Unlimiting mind: The radically experiential psychology of Buddhism.* Somerville, MA: Wisdom.

Öst, L. G. (2008). Efficacy of the third wave of behavioral therapies: A systematic review and meta-analysis. *Behaviour Research and Therapy, 46,* 296–321.

Pace, T. W., Negi, L. T., Adame, D. D., Cole, S. P., Sivilli, T. I., Brown, T. D., et al. (2009). Effect of compassion meditation on neuroendocrine, innate immune and behavioral responses to psychosocial stress. *Psychoneuroendocrinology, 34*(1), 87–98.

Pagnoni, G., & Cekic, M. (2007). Age effects on gray matter volume and attentional performance in Zen meditation. *Neurobiology of Aging, 28,* 1623–1627.

Pani, L., Porcella, A., & Gessa, G. L. (2000). The role of stress in the pathophysiology of the dopaminergic system. *Molecular Psychiatry, 5,* 14–21.

Panksepp, J. (1994). The basics of basic emotion. In P. Ekman & R. J. Davidson (Eds.), *The nature of emotion* (pp. 20–24). New York: Oxford University Press.

Panksepp, J. (1998). The periconscious substrates of consciousness: Affective states and the evolutionary origins of the self. *Journal of Consciousness Studies, 5*(5–6), 566–582.

Pauley, G., & McPherson, S. (2010). The experience and meaning of compassion and self-compassion for individuals with depression or anxiety. *Psychology and Psychotherapy: Theory, Research and Practice, 83*(2), 129–143.

Pelden, K. (2007). The nectar of Manjushri's speech: A detailed commentary on Shantideva's Way of the Bodhisattva (Padmakara Translation Group, Trans.). Boston: Shambhala.

Posner, M. I., & Petersen, S. E. (1990). The attention system of the human brain. *Annual Review of Neuroscience, 13*, 25–42.

Posner, M. I., & Rothbart, M. K. (2007). Research on attention networks as a model for the integration of psychological science. *Annual Review of Psychology, 58*, 1–23.

Rahula, W. (1959/1974). *What the Buddha taught.* New York: Grove Press.

Ramel, W., Goldin, P. R., Carmona, P. E., & McQuaid, J. R. (2004). The effects of mindfulness meditation on cognitive processes and affect in patients with past depression. *Cognitive Therapy and Research, 28*, 433–455.

Ramnero, J., & Torneke, N. (2008). *The ABCs of human behavior: Behavioral principles for the practicing clinician.* Oakland, CA: New Harbinger.

Rapgay, L., & Bystrisky, A. (2009). Classical mindfulness. *Annals of the New York Academy of Sciences, 1172*, 148–162.

Reale, G. (1987). *A history of ancient philosophy: From the origins to Socrates* (Vol. 1). Albany: State University of New York Press.

Rector, N. A., Bagby, R. M., Segal, Z. V., Joffe, R. T., & Levitt, A. (2000). Self-criticism and dependency in depressed patients treated with cognitive therapy or pharmacotherapy. *Cognitive Therapy and Research, 24*, 571–584.

Reibel, D. K., Greeson, J. M., Brainard, G. C., & Rosenzweig, S. (2001). Mindfulness-based stress reduction and health-related quality of life in a heterogeneous patient population. *General Hospital Psychiatry, 23*(4), 183–192.

Roemer, L., & Orsillo, S. M. (2002). Expanding our conceptualization of and treatment for generalized anxiety disorder: Integrating mindfulness/acceptance-based approaches with existing cognitive behavioral models. *Clinical Psychology Science and Practice, 9*, 54–68.

Roemer, L., & Orsillo, S. M. (2007). An open trial of an acceptance-based behavior therapy for generalized anxiety disorder. *Behavior Therapy, 38*(1), 72–85.

Roemer, L., & Orsillo, S. M. (2009). *Mindfulness- and acceptance-based behavioral therapies in practice.* New York: Guilford Press.

Roemer, L., Orsillo, S. M., & Salters-Pedneault, K. (2008). Efficacy of an acceptance-based behavior therapy for generalized anxiety disorder: Evaluation in a randomized controlled trial. *Journal of Consulting and Clinical Psychology, 76*(6), 1083-1089.

Ruiz, F. J. (2010). A review of acceptance and commitment therapy (ACT) empirical evidence: Correlational, experimental psychopathology, component and outcome studies. *International Journal of Psychology and Psychological Therapy, 10*, 125–162.

Sachs-Ericsson, N., Verona, E., Joiner, T., & Preacher, J. K. (2006). Parental verbal abuse and the mediating role of self-criticism in adult internalizing disorders. *Journal of Affective Disorders, 93*, 71–78.

Sahdra, B. K., MacLean, K. A., Ferrer, E., Shaver, P. R., Rosenberg, E. L., Jacobs, T. L., et al. (2011). Enhanced response inhibition during intensive meditation training predicts improvements in self-reported adaptive socio-emotional functioning. *Emotion, 11*(2), 299–312.

Salkovskis, P. M., Clark, D. M., Hackmann, A., Wells, A., & Gelder, M. G. (1999). An experimental investigation of the role of safety-seeking behaviours in the maintenance of panic disorder with agoraphobia. *Behaviour Research and Therapy, 37*(6), 559–574.

Salters-Pedneault, K., Tull, M. T., & Roemer, L. (2004). The role of avoidance of emotional material in the anxiety disorders. *Applied and Preventive Psychology, 11*, 95–114.

Santideva. (1997). The way of the bodhisattva (Padmakara Translation Group, Trans.). Boston: Shambhala.

Sears, R., Tirch, D., & Denton, R. (2011). *Mindfulness in clinical practice.* Sarasota, FL: Professional Resources Exchange.

Sedlmeier, P., Eberth, J., Schwarz, M., Zimmermann, D., Haarig, F., Jaeger, S., & Kunze, S. (2012). The psychological effects of meditation: A meta-analysis. *Psychological Bulletin, 138*(6), 1139-1171.

Segal, Z. V., Williams, J. M. G., & Teasdale, J. D. (2002). *Mindfulness-based cognitive therapy for depression: A new approach to preventing relapse.* New York: Guilford Press.

Segal, Z. V., Williams, J. M. G., & Teasdale, J. D. (2012). *Mindfulness-based cognitive therapy for depression* (2nd ed.). New York: Guilford Press.

Shallcross, A. J., Troy, A. S., Boland, M., & Mauss, I. B. (2010). Let it be: Accepting negative emotional experiences predicts decreased negative affect and depressive symptoms. *Behaviour Research and Therapy, 48*(9), 921–929.

Shambhala dictionary of Buddhism and Zen. (1991). Boston: Shambhala.

Shantideva. (1997). *A guide to the Bodhisattva's way of life* (V. A. Wallace & B. A. Wallace, Trans.). Ithaca, NY: Snow Lion.

Shapiro, S. L., Astin, J. A., Bishop, S. R., & Cordova, M. (2005). Mindfulness-based stress reduction for health care professionals: Results from a randomized trial. *International Journal of Stress Management, 12*, 164–176.

Shapiro, S. L., & Schwartz, G. E. (2000). Intentional systemic mindfulness: An integrative model for self-regulation and health. *Advances in Mind–Body Medicine, 16*, 128–134.

Shepherd, D. A., & Cardon, M. S. (2009). Negative emotional reactions to project failure and the self-compassion to learn from the experience. *Journal of Management Studies, 46*(6), 923–949.

Siegel, D. J. (2007a). *The mindful brain.* New York: Norton.

Siegel, D. J. (2007b). Mindfulness training and neural integration: Differentiation of distinct streams of awareness and the cultivation of wellbeing. *Social Cognitive and Affective Neuroscience, 2*, 259–263.

Siegel, D. J. (2009). Mindful awareness, mindsight, and neural integration. *The Humanistic Psychologist, 37*, 137–158.

Siegel, R. D., Germer, C. K., & Olendzki, A. (2009). Mindfulness: What is it? Where did it come from? In F. Didonna (Ed.), *Clinical handbook of mindfulness* (pp. 17–35). New York: Springer.

Skinner, B. F. (1953). *Science and human behavior.* New York: Free Press.

Skinner, B. F. (1974). *About behaviourism.* New York: Random House Digital.

Snyder, C. R., Ilardi, S. S., Cheavens, J., Michael, S. T., Yamhure, L., & Sympson, S. (2000). The role of hope in cognitive-behavior therapies. *Cognitive Therapy and Research, 24,* 747–762.

Sopa, G. L., & Newman, B. (2008). *Steps on the path to enlightenment: A commentary on Tsong-kha-pa's Lamrim Chenmo: Vol. 3. The way of the bodhisattva.* Somerville, MA: Wisdom.

Stewart, I., Villatte, J., & McHugh, L. (2012). Approaches to the self. In L. McHugh & I. Stewart (Eds.), *The self and perspective taking: Contributions and applications from modern behavioral science* (pp. 3–36). Oakland, CA: New Harbinger.

Succito, A. (2010). *Turning the wheel of truth: Commentary on the Buddha's first teaching.* Boston: Shambhala.

Surrey, J. L. (2005). Relational psychotherapy, relational mindfulness. In C. K. Germer, R. D. Siegel, & P. R. Fulton (Eds.), *Mindfulness and psychotherapy* (pp. 91–110). New York: Guilford Press.

Suzuki, S. (1970). *Zen mind, beginner's mind.* Boston: Weatherhill Press.

Tang, Y. Y., Ma, Y., Fan, Y., Feng, H., Wang, J., Feng, S., et al. (2009). Central and autonomic nervous system interaction is altered by short-term meditation. *Proceedings of the National Academy of Sciences, 106,* 8865–8870.

Tangney, J. P. (1995). Shame and guilt in interpersonal relationships. In J. P. Tangney & K. W. Fischer (Eds.), *Self-conscious emotions: The psychology of shame, guilt, embarrassment, and pride* (pp. 114–139). New York: Guilford Press.

Teasdale, J. D. (1999). Emotional processing, three modes of mind and the prevention of relapse and depression. *Behaviour Research and Therapy, 37*(Suppl.), S53–S77.

Teasdale, J. D., & Chaskalson, M. (2011). How does mindfulness transform suffering?: I. The nature and origins of dukkha. *Contemporary Buddhism, 12*(1), 89–102.

Teasdale, J. D., Moore, R. G., Hayhurst, H., Pope, M., Williams, S., & Segal, Z. V. (2002). Metacognitive awareness and prevention of relapse in depression: Empirical evidence. *Journal of Consulting and Clinical Psychology, 70,* 275–287.

Teasdale, J. D., Segal, Z. V., & Williams, J. M. G. (2003). Mindfulness training and problem formulation. *Clinical Psychology, 10,* 157–160.

Teasdale, J. D., Segal, Z. V., Williams, J. M. G., & Mark, G. (1995). How does cognitive therapy prevent depressive relapse and why should attentional control (mindfulness) training help? *Behaviour Research and Therapy, 33,* 25–39.

Terry, M. L., & Leary, M. R. (2011). Self-compassion, self-regulation, and health. *Self and Identity, 10*(3), 352–362.

Thera, N. (1962). *The heart of Buddhist meditation.* New York: Samuel Weiser.

Thera, S. (1998). *The way of mindfulness: The Satipatthana Sutta and its commentary.* Kandy, Sri Lanka: Buddhist Publication Society.

Thompson, B. L., & Waltz, J. (2008). Self-compassion and PTSD symptom severity. *Journal of Traumatic Stress, 21,* 556–558.

Thurman, R. (1997). *Essential Tibetan Buddhism.* Edison, NJ: Castle Books.

Tirch, D. D. (2010). Mindfulness as a context for the cultivation of compassion. *International Journal of Cognitive Therapy, 3*(2), 113–123.

Tirch, D. D. (2012). *The compassionate mind approach to overcoming anxiety: Using compassion focused therapy.* London: Constable & Robinson.

Tirch, D. D., & Amodio, R. (2006). Beyond mindfulness and posttraumatic stress disorder. In M. G. T. Kwee, K. J. Gergen, & F. Koshikawa (Eds.), *Horizons in Buddhist psychology* (pp. 101–118). Taos, NM: Taos Institute Publications.

Tirch, D. [D.], & Gilbert, P. (2014). Compassion-focused therapy. In N. C. Thoma & D. McKay (Eds.), *Working with emotion in cognitive-behavioral therapy: Techniques for clinical practice* (pp. 59–79). New York: Guilford Press.

Tirch, D. [D.], Schoendorff, B., & Silberstein, L. R. (2014). *The ACT practitioner's guide to the science of compassion: Tools for fostering psychological flexibility.* Oakland: CA: New Harbinger.

Toneatto, T., Vettese, L., & Nguyen, L. (2007). The role of mindfulness in the cognitive-behavioural treatment of problem gambling. *Journal of Gambling Issues, 19,* 91–100.

Törneke, N. (2010). *Learning RFT: An introduction to relational frame theory and its clinical application.* Oakland, CA: New Harbinger.

Treadway, M. T., & Lazar, M. T. (2009). The neurobiology of mindfulness. In F. Diodonna (Ed.), *Clinical handbook of mindfulness* (pp. 45–58). New York: Springer.

Treanor, M. (2011). The potential impact of mindfulness on exposure and extinction learning in anxiety disorders. *Clinical Psychology Review, 31,* 617–625.

Trungpa, C. (2005). *The sanity we are born with.* Boston: Shambhala.

Tsong-Kha-Pa. (2002). *Lam Rim Chen Mo: The great treatise on the stages of the path to enlightenment* (Vol. 3; Lamrim Chenmo Translation Committee, Trans.). Ithaca, NY: Snow Lion.

Valentine, E., & Sweet, P. (1999). Meditation and attention: A comparison of the effects of concentrative and mindfulness meditation on sustained attention. *Mental Health, Religion and Culture, 2,* 59–70.

van den Hurk, P. A., Giommi, F., Gielen, S. C., Speckens, A. E., & Barendregt, H. P. (2010). Greater efficiency in attentional processing related to mindfulness meditation. *Quarterly Journal of Experimental Psychology, 63,* 1168–1180.

Varela, F. J. (1996). Neurophenomenology: A methodological remedy for the hard problem. *Journal of Consciousness Studies, 3*(4), 330–349.

Varela, F. [J.] (1997). The specious present: A neurophenomenlogy of time consciousness. In J. Petitot, F. J.Varela, J.-M. Roy, & B. Pachoud (Eds.), *Naturalizing phenomenology: Issues in contemporary phenomenology and cognitive science* (pp. 266–316). Stanford, CA: Stanford University Press.

Varela, F. [J.] (2000). Steps to a science of inter-being. In G. Watson, S., Batchelor, & G. Claxton (Eds.), *The psychology of awakening: Buddhism, science, and our day-to-day lives* (pp. 71–89). Newbury Port, MA: Weiser Books.

Villagran, M., Goldsmith, J., Wittenberg-Lyles, E., & Baldwin, P. (2010). Creating COMFORT: A communication-based model for breaking bad news. *Communication Education, 59*(3), 220–234.

Voegelin, E. (1978). *Anamnesis* (G. Niemeyer, Trans. & Ed.). Notre Dame, IN: University of Notre Dame Press. (Originally published 1966)

Vujanovic, A. A., Zvolensky, M. J., Bernstein, A., Feldner, M. T., & McLeish, A. C. (2007). A test of the interactive effects of anxiety sensitivity and mindfulness in the prediction of anxious arousal, agoraphobic cognitions, and body vigilance. *Behaviour Research and Therapy, 45*, 1393–1400.

Wachs, K., & Cordova, J. V. (2007). Mindful relating: Exploring mindfulness and emotion repertoires in intimate relationships. *Journal of Marital and Family Therapy, 33*, 464–481.

Wallace, B. A. (2003). Introduction: Buddhism and science—Breaking down the barriers. In B. A. Wallace (Ed.), *Buddhism and science: Breaking new ground* (pp. 1–30). New York: Columbia University Press.

Wallace, B. A. (2011). A Buddhist view of free will: Beyond determinism and indeterminism. *Journal of Consciousness Studies, 18*(3–4), 17–33.

Wallace, B. A., & Shapiro, S. L. (2006). Mental balance and well-being: Building bridges between Buddhism and Western psychology. *American Psychologist, 61*(7), 690–701.

Wang, S. (2005). A conceptual framework for integrating research related to the physiology of compassion and the wisdom of Buddhist teachings. In P. Gilbert (Ed.), *Compassion: Conceptualisations, research and use in psychotherapy* (pp. 75–101). New York: Routledge.

Way, B. M., Creswell, J. D., Eisenberger, N. I., & Lieberman, M. D. (2010). Dispositional mindfulness and depressive symptomatology: Correlations with limbic and self-referential neural activity during rest. *Emotion, 10*, 12–24.

Webster's new world dictionary (3rd college ed.). (1988). New York: Websters New World

Wegner, D. M., Schneider, D. J., Carter, S. R., & White, T. L. (1987). Paradoxical effects of thought suppression. *Journal of Personality and Social Psychology, 53*, 5–13.

Welford, M. (2010). A compassion focused approach to anxiety disorders. *International Journal of Cognitive Therapy, 3*, 124–140.

Welford, M. (2012). *The compassionate mind approach to building self-confidence: Using compassion focused therapy.* London: Constable & Robinson.

Wells, A. (1995). Meta-cognition and worry: A cognitive model of generalized anxiety disorder. *Behavioural and Cognitive Psychotherapy, 23*(3), 301–320.

Wenzlaff, R. M., & Wegner, D. M. (2000). Thought suppression. *Annual Review of Psychology, 51*, 59–91.

White, K. S., Brown, T. A., Somers, T. J., & Barlow, D. H. (2006). Avoidance behavior in panic disorder: The moderating influence of perceived control. *Behaviour Research and Therapy, 44*, 147–157.

Wiist, W. H., Sullivan, B. M., George, D. M., & Wayment, H. A. (2012). Buddhists' religious and health practices. *Journal of Religion and Health, 51*, 132–147.

Williams, J. C., & Lynn, S. J. (2011). Acceptance: An historical and conceptual review. *Imagination, Cognition, and Personality, 30*(1), 5–56.

Williams, J. M. G. (2010). Mindfulness and psychological process. *Emotion, 10*, 1–7.

Wilson, D. S. (2004). What is wrong with absolute individual fitness? *Trends in Ecology and Evolution, 19*, 245–248.

Wilson, D. S. (2007). *Evolution for everyone: How Darwin's theory can change the way we think about our lives.* New York: Delcacort Press.

Wilson, D. S., Hayes, S. C., Biglan, A., & Embry, D. D. (2014). Evolving the future: Toward a science of intentional change. *Behavioral and Brain Sciences, 37*(4), 395–416.

Wilson, K. G., & DuFrene, T. (2009). *Mindfulness for two: An acceptance and commitment therapy approach to mindfulness in psychotherapy.* Oakland, CA: New Harbinger.

Wood, J. T. (2004). Buddhist influences on teaching and writing. *Journal of Communication and Religion, 27*, 32–39.

Woolfolk, R. L. (1998). *The cure of souls: Science, values, and psychotherapy.* San Francisco: Jossey-Bass.

Wupperman, P., Marlatt, G. A., Cunningham, A., Bowen, S., Berking, M., Mulvihill-Rivera, N., et al. (2012). Mindfulness and modification therapy for behavioral dysregulation: results from a pilot study targeting alcohol use and aggression in women. *Journal of Clinical Psychology, 68*(1), 50–66.

Yeshe, L. T., & Ribush, N. (2000). *Make your mind an ocean—Aspects of Buddhist psychology.* Geylang, Singapore: Amitabha Buddhist Centre.

Young, J. D. E., & Taylor, E. (1998). Meditation as a voluntary hypometabolic state of biological estivation. *Physiology, 13*(3), 149–153.

Zajonc, R. B. (1984). On the primacy of affect. *American Psychologist, 39*, 117–123.

Zeidan, F., Johnson, S. K., Gordon, N. S., & Goolkasian, P. (2010). Effects of brief and sham mindfulness meditation on mood and cardiovascular variables. *Journal of Alternative and Complementary Medicine, 16*(8), 867–873.

Zuroff, D. C., Mongrain, M., & Santor, D. A. (2004). Conceptualizing and measuring personality vulnerability to depression: Comment on Coyne and Whiffen (1995). *Psychological Bulletin, 130*(3), 489.

Index

Page numbers in italic denote a figure or table.

255